The DMSO
Handbook
for Doctors

The DMSO Handbook for Doctors

Archie H. Scott

iUniverse, Inc.
Bloomington

THE DMSO HANDBOOK FOR DOCTORS

iUniverse books may be ordered through booksellers or by contacting:

iUniverse
1663 Liberty Drive
Bloomington, IN 47403
www.iuniverse.com
1-800-Authors (1-800-288-4677)

ISBN: 978-1-4759-9792-7 (sc)
ISBN: 978-1-4759-9793-4 (ebk)

Library of Congress Control Number: 2013912102

Printed in the United States of America

iUniverse rev. date: 07/02/2013

Contents

Acknowledgements

There are many people who have provided information and encouragement to the author over the years that he has been involved in research and investigation of DMSO. Stanley Jacob M.D., the father of DMSO and my mentor, provided me much early information on DMSO and was the person most responsible for getting me interested in DMSO and medical research and treatment in general.

Frank Cousineau and Lorraine Rosenthal of the Cancer Control Society have always given information and encouragement.

Others who have had a major influence either on this book or on my experience with DMSO or health information or products in general include Linda Walton, Dr. Veronika Voss, Dr. Carolyn Goldman, Irving Schultz, Gary Schultz, Irving Schaeffner MD, Marjorie Ward, Leona Reams, Travis Thomas, and Evelyn Jackson.

We would also like to thank Jessica "Jay" Yurick for her typing and computer skills.

Ron Bronson proved to be an excellent editor with a great ability to spot errors.

Two organizations also deserve recognition for what they have done for medical and health research and information. These are the New York Academy of Sciences and The Cancer Control Society. Both of these organizations are known for providing honest, reliable information.

Forewords

We have known Archie Scott since 1976. He did not introduce us to DMSO, but he did provide practical knowledge in how to use DMSO to improve daily life. Further, he provided the inspiration to share the knowledge with family, friends and colleagues.

Over the years since we met, we have increased our knowledge exponentially from discussions and collaboration with Archie. His knowledge of the compound is tremendous. His practical applications in the clinical setting are well-known to physicians in the United States and Mexico, plus numerous other countries around the globe. Archie is among the top two or three world-wide sources for valuable, accurate information related to DMSO, its properties, its uses and its applications in the clinic, home and work place.

This volume is designed to be of benefit to clinician, researcher and ultimate consumer. It contains the references necessary to satisfy the medical professional and technical information so the practicing physician can administer DMSO to his patients. Every emergency room should have this book in order to save lives from a wide variety of medical conditions. The use of DMSO in veterinarian medicine is well-known and accepted. It is time for human medicine to adopt its near miraculous benefits without the *negative effects* associated with toxic and potentially fatal pharmaceutical products.

A bottle of DMSO should be in the locker room of every athletic facility and *First Aid Kit* of every athletic Coach and Trainer. This book should be included with the bottle of DMSO.

This book is also written so the non-professional can read it and benefit from the safe and effective properties of DMSO. It is organized in a logical format to make it easy to use as a convenient and accessible reference.

Archie Scott has provided a very valuable benefit to mankind with the publication of this book. His *raison d'etre* is to alleviate suffering and advance scientific knowledge. We believe this compact volume will do both.

Frank Cousineau
President, Life Support
President, Cancer Control Society
President, International Association
of Cancer Victors and Friends
May 2013

Chapter 1

Introduction

Dimethyl sulfoxide, commonly called DMSO, has been described by its supporters (nearly everyone who has ever used it) as a true medical miracle. It has been used in the treatment of hundreds of ailments that afflict people throughout the world. In fact, by itself, or in combination with other medications, DMSO has proven useful in the treatment of practically every medical problem known.

What is DMSO? It is a natural chemical compound derived from trees as a by-product from the manufacturing of paper. It is composed of two methyl groups (CH3) and a sulfur and an oxygen atom. It was first synthesized by a Russian chemist, Alexander Zaytsev, in 1866. For over eighty years DMSO was basically ignored. During the late 1940s industrial chemists started investigating the solvent capabilities of DMSO. Improved solvents were needed, and there was interest in utilizing tree derived waste products.

Commercial development of DMSO was started in the 1950s. Crown Zellerbach, a large American paper manufacturing company, started producing DMSO during this time and became the largest producer of DMSO in the world. At this time Robert J. Herschler was the supervisor of applications research in the chemical products division of the Crown Zellerbach plant in Camas, Washington, which is across the Columbia River from Oregon Health Sciences University. As a chemist Mr. Herschler conducted research on DMSO and other tree derived chemicals.

Stanley W. Jacob, M.D. was head of the organ transplant team at the University of Oregon Medical School which is now called Oregon Health Sciences University. He needed a way to preserve transplant organs at a low temperature without the formation of ice crystals. Various products and procedures were tried without success. Before DMSO there was no way to preserve organs without the formation of ice crystals which killed the tissue.

In 1961 Dr. Jacob and Robert Herschler met for the first time, and Dr. Jacob was introduced to the anti-freeze capabilities of DMSO. The preservation of transplant organs is still one of the many uses of DMSO. While 100% DMSO will freeze at 66 degrees, a 50% mixture of DMSO and water will not freeze at temperatures far below the freezing point of straight water.

Dr. Jacob soon discovered that DMSO had many other properties that would later prove to make DMSO one of the most important medical products ever discovered. Just a few of these properties, or even one by itself, could make DMSO an important product in the treatment of a wide variety of conditions. When all these properties are combined in one substance, we have a truly amazing product.

DMSO has been described by Dr. Jacob as a new medical principle. It is a substance that is totally strange to medical science. Its mode of action is not completely understood, and it is used to treat some ailments that have long been considered as untreatable. Also, because of its distinctive odor, it is very difficult to conduct double blind studies with DMSO. However, it is always possible to have studies involving DMSO where the results are compared to current treatment. As an example, if a disease at a certain stage has an expected mortality rate of 80% within one year, and there is a 10% mortality rate for those treated with DMSO, it shows that DMSO is a successful treatment. If the mortality rate stays in the 80 % range, it shows no improvement.

Methylsulfonylmethane, commonly called MSM, is a product that is derived from DMSO. MSM has many of the properties of DMSO, but is generally regarded as a food supplement. It has not been subject to the medical studies of DMSO and is not considered to be as effective as DMSO in treating most ailments. However, it also does not cause the patient to have the garlic-like DMSO breath.

DMSO is one of the most powerful free radical scavengers known. Free radicals are unstable charged molecular fragments that attack other molecules causing severe damage to cells throughout the body. This disrupts the normal functioning of various organs in the body. Free radical damage is usually slow and accumulates over the years. Eventually this can lead to such ailments as cancer and arthritis. It can also lead to premature aging. It is possible that the regular use of DMSO may completely prevent some serious ailments.

Another important action of DMSO is its immune normalizing effect. This makes DMSO important in the treatment of autoimmune diseases and can also help the natural immune system fight off various infectious and contagious diseases.

DMSO also passes through the skin and other cellular membranes of the body. This is the reason that the application of a small amount of DMSO applied topically to the skin can cause a garlic like breath odor. DMSO is one of the few products that are able to cross the blood brain barrier. It is also able to take other products that normally do not cross this barrier with it. This could make DMSO valuable in the treatment of many brain problems.

Another important action of DMSO is it is a vasodilator. This can increase blood flow, allowing blood to more easily reach areas where damage may have occurred. Often an injury causes decreased blood flow to the injury site, and some of the damage is caused by the lack of blood to the area after the injury, and not just the injury itself.

In many cases DMSO is used to treat one problem, and it ends up helping a completely unrelated health problem. It is hoped that this book will lead more doctors both in the United States and other countries around the world to try DMSO, especially in treating their more difficult cases where nothing else seems to help.

Chapter 2

Amyloidosis

Amyloidosis is a disease characterized by amyloid proteins abnormally deposited in various tissues in the body. A protein is amyloid if due to an alteration in its secondary structure, it takes on an aggregated insoluble form similar to the beta-pleated sheet.

Approximately 60 different amyloid proteins have been identified, and at least 36 have been found to be involved in some way with a human disease.

Amyloidosis can be very difficult to diagnose especially in the early stages. Symptoms vary widely depending upon where in the body the amyloid deposits accumulate.

Many patients go undiagnosed. Amyloidosis can affect so many internal organs, and the symptoms can resemble so many other ailments that other problems are often suspected.

Amyloidosis can be localized or systemic. The localized form only affects one organ or one part of the body. It does no damage to the rest of the body. Two common conditions associated with localized amyloidosis are Type 2 diabetes where the amyloid protein builds up in the pancreas and Alzheimer's where the amyloid proteins build up in the brain. The next chapter offers more details on the amyloid proteins of Alzheimer's.

Systemic amyloidosis can cause damage to any organ in the body. Often a variety of unrelated organs are involved, and death can be caused by toxic activity in any of these organs.

The heart is often involved, and there can be a wide variety of symptoms in the heart ranging from arrhythmia and irregular heartbeat to congestive heart failure. The respiratory tract can be affected. The spleen can enlarge and sometimes rupture. The gastrointestinal tract is sometimes affected causing diarrhea, vomiting, and hemorrhaging.

Conventional treatment for amyloidosis has consisted mostly of steroids and chemotherapy. Stem cell transplants are also sometimes done. All of these treatments have usually resulted in limited success.

An important mouse study involving the use of DSMO was conducted by Mordechai Ravid, Igal Kedar, M. Greenwald, and Ezra Sohar at the Sachler School of Medicine, Tel Aviv University in Israel. Amyloidosis was induced in these mice by injecting them daily for 18 days with vitamin-free casein. They were then studied for the following 60 days until they were killed and autopsied.

The urine of the mice treated with DMSO showed broken up amyloid fibrils starting shortly after the start of DMSO treatment. When the DMSO treated mice were autopsied their livers were completely free of amyloid deposits. The livers of the control mice that were not treated with DSMO were loaded with amyloid. This study showed that DMSO dissolved the amyloid protein.

Other studies have shown mixed results. However, no studies have shown any adverse reactions when treating amyloidosis with DMSO. Therefore, there is no reason not to treat all cases of amyloidosis with DMSO. This does not mean that DMSO should be the only treatment. DMSO could be combined with any other treatment that may be used allowing such other treatment to work more effectively.

Chapter 3

Alzheimer's and other Dementia

Dementia of various types, especially Alzheimer's, has become increasingly more of a problem as the general population ages. DMSO would logically be expected to help with all forms of dementia. In the test tube DMSO causes immature brain cells to mature. It also increases blood flow in the brain.

As a person ages circulation usually gradually becomes impaired. This can result in a lack of oxygen and nutrients to the brain. With a reduced amount of oxygen and nutrients brain cells can be injured or killed. DMSO can prevent this from happening. DMSO also helps the neurons in the brain to communicate with each other. All of this helps enable the person to retain mental capabilities into advanced age.

This writer had a friend who died at the age of 101. She was a strong advocate of DMSO and had used it regularly for over 30 years. When she was 101 she showed no sign of mental decline. She was an authority on the Bible and had a general intelligence level that was better than the average 30 year old. No one knows how well her mind would have worked without the DMSO, but it is probable that her superior mind at such an advanced age was at least partially due to DMSO.

One of the most important uses of DMSO is in the treatment of patients with Alzheimer's. DMSO has been shown to dissolve amyloids, the proteins that occur in the brain lesions of patients with Alzheimer's. It has now become generally accepted that the beta amyloid protein is involved in the development and progression of Alzheimer's. Large numbers of amyloid plaques and tangles are always present in confirmed cases of Alzheimer's and the extent of this amyloid corresponds closely with the amount of dementia. A thorough description of the amyloid proteins is contained in a 1989 article in Microbiology of Aging.[1]

What causes a normal protein to become amyloidgenic? There are several theories that are possible. One of the most probable is that some form of inflammation could cause damage to a normal protein. Once an abnormal process starts the process can replicate and become more abnormal.

Professor Jeffrey Kelly of Scripps Research Institute has put forth the theory that inflammation could be the start of a process that ultimately leads to Alzheimer's. Normal brain cells can be disrupted as a result of inflammation. and this could cause amyloid beta proteins in the brain to misfold. According to Kelly the inflammation process might occur years before the onset of Alzheimer's and could be caused by a variety of infections.

To test his theory Kelly and colleagues checked the brains of Alzheimer's victims and found evidence of a substance called atheronals. Atheronals have only recently been discovered and refer to the way ozone reacts with normal metabolites to produce toxic compounds during inflammatory processes taking place in the body.

Kelly and his associates also performed test tube experiments and found that atheronals and lipid oxidation products can greatly accelerate the misfolding of amyloid beta proteins. Kelly admits that it will be difficult to prove his theory, but it is an interesting and realistic idea.

The results of a study involving the use of DMSO in the treatment of patients with Alzheimer's was presented at the Fourth International Conference on Alzheimer's Disease and Related Disorders.[2] In this study 18 patients with probable Alzheimer's were treated with DMSO and tested regularly for nine months.

Great improvements were noted in these patients after only three months of treatment. The improvement was especially noticeable after six months of treatment. Efficacy of treatment was obtained from the results of neurological and neuropsychological testing that showed improvement in memory, concentration, and communication. Disorientation in time and space also decreased greatly.

Based on the previous examples it is probable that everyone suffering from Alzheimer's or any other form of dementia should be treated with DMSO. Treatment should be started as soon as major decline is noted in the patient. Improvement is more dramatic with early stage patients. If the condition has been allowed to progress beyond a certain point it can be impossible to reverse the damage. Those that really desire to maintain good mental health into old age should probably be on DMSO before any decline in mental health is noticed.

[1.] Caputa, Claudio B. and Andre I. Salama. The Amyloid Proteins of Alzheimer's Disease as Potential Targets for Drug Therapy, Microbiology of Aging Volume 10, pp451-461.

[2.] Goppa, S. A. New Possibilities in the Treatment of Patients with Alzheimer's Disease. Department of Neurology and Neurosurgery, Medical University, Kisheiner, Moldova.

Chapter 4

Arthritis

Over 21 million Americans suffer from arthritis according to the Arthritis Foundation. This arthritis can be relatively mild with minor pain some of the time or very severe with major pain and loss of mobility. Arthritis is the number one cause of disability for people over 65.

Conventional medical treatment uses a dangerous combination of painkillers whose purpose is only to stop the pain from the arthritis. Medication such as aspirin, cortisone, and nonsteroidal anti-inflammatory drugs do not prevent or correct the problem. They do reduce pain, but can be very detrimental to the health of the patient, especially if taken for a long period of time.

Non-steroidal anti-inflammatory drugs can be especially harmful to the patient's joints. NSAIDs block the enzymes that help produce inflammatory compounds. However, they also inhibit the action of enzymes that help produce cartilage. Therefore, the patient will probably have some pain relief while taking the NSAIDs while at the same time they may be actually making the arthritic process worse.

How about other more natural medications? Many patients have reported positive effects with glucosamine sulfate. Even more have reported good results from using MSM. Neither of these products seems to produce negative side effects while at the same time there is often greatly reduced pain. A number of medical studies have shown low levels of sulfur in arthritic joints. This would lead to the probability that lack of sulfur is a factor in osteoarthritis.

Most people with arthritis that visit hot spring health resorts report positive results. The water in these hot springs usually contains a large amount of natural sulfur. While the hot water may also be of benefit, the most important healing aspect of these hot springs is most likely the sulfur in the water.

There have been arthritis clinics using injections of DMSO that have claimed results in three days. These have not generally been reliable. It takes more than three days to completely treat arthritis and obtain lasting results. However, there are cases where immediate temporary relief is obtained.

There is general agreement among doctors who have treated arthritis patients and the patients themselves that DMSO is the best treatment for arthritis, whether it is osteoarthritis or rheumatoid arthritis. This treatment may be straight DMSO, or DMSO combined with other products. Also, the DMSO may be applied topically to the affected area, injected, or taken by mouth.

When DMSO was first used, most arthritis patients were treated topically with DMSO applied to the affected area. There are now topical lotions that contain DMSO and other products in combination that are even more effective than straight DMSO.

An example of a patient who got immediate results was a 67 year-old man who could not move his finger. A lotion containing DMSO and capsicum pepper was applied to this man's finger. A few minutes later he was moving his finger. He was amazed and kept moving the finger. His wife watched him move the finger and while watching asked: "Jack, can you really move that finger?" His answer was: "Yes, don't you see it moving?"

DMSO does several things to help improve arthritis and does not have the negative side effects of many other medications such as the NSAIDs. First DMSO greatly reduces the pain and muscle spasms around arthritic joints. It improves blood flow which helps bring needed nutrients to the damaged area. It provides biologically available sulfur to the damaged joint. DMSO also reduces inflammation.

It is my opinion that the most important factor about DMSO in the treatment of arthritis is the fact that DMSO is the most potent free radical scavenger known. Free radicals have been implicated as the leading or one of the leading causes of many degenerative ailments. It is logical that free radicals do play a role in both rheumatoid and osteoarthritis.

Free radical activity as a cause of arthritis was simply a logical theory for a period of time and to my knowledge no study of the free radical activity in arthritis has been done in the United States. However, a very good private study was performed in Brazil.

The study in Brazil involved 30 patients with the purpose of confirming the relationship between free radical synthesis and arthritis. This study was conducted at Centro Internacional de Medicina Preventia in Sao Paulo, Brazil. Even though osteoarthritis is a degenerative disease and rheumatoid arthritis is considered to be an autoimmune disease, they have certain things in common. The symptoms are similar, and both can severely cripple the patient.

This clinic regularly used DMSO to treat arthritis patients, and it was known that the treatment was of great benefit to the patient. However, this study was to verify that DMSO not only provided clinical improvement, but also reduced the formation of free radicals.

The patients chosen were regular patients at the clinic. Fifteen of the patients had osteoarthritis and 15 had rheumatoid arthritis. The HLB (Heiton-La Garde-Bradford) test which measures the reactive oxygen toxic species was used to test for free radical production.

The treatment used was the same as had been used on all arthritis patients for the previous five years. For this study 5ccs of DMSO were used along with B complex, vitamin C and magnesium sulfate. An infusion was given two times a week for five weeks, then once a month for 18 months. These patients were tested for free radicals before the study started, immediately after a DMSO infusion, and again after the study was completed. The results showed a 66% decrease in free radical production after DMSO administration. Following completion of the study there was a 52% decrease in free radical production from the level at the beginning.

With this protocol they have had good clinical improvement of symptoms in over 85% of the patients with osteoarthritis and 77% of the patients with rheumatoid arthritis. These results were long lasting and obtained without the use of any steroidal or non-steroidal anti-inflammatory drugs.

Nearly all the arthritis patients treated with DMSO that this writer is familiar with have noted improvement in both relief of pain and increased range of motion. One patient, who is now 63 years-old, was a high school football and basketball player. He later ran marathons (26 miles races) for over 20 years. He first noticed increasing pain in his knees and hips. Later he said he had pain everywhere. His doctor gave him prescriptions for more powerful pain killers and an injection of cortisone. He was told that he should be on pain killers for the rest of his life.

This man knew that the medications were harming his body, but he also wanted relief of pain. He was finally told to try more natural treatments. He found that there was slight improvement when he used glucosamine sulfate. One year later he was introduced to DMSO. A 90% solution of DMSO was applied to his knees every day, and he also drank DMSO—one teaspoonful every day in four ounces of juice. He immediately started to feel better and also noted increased energy. Two years later this man has little pain and says that he can also think more clearly.

Doctors who have treated arthritic patients with DMSO have recommended various combinations and methods of treatment. Some prefer topical application. Others prefer to have the patient drink the DMSO in juice or water. If the patient is taking many powerful medications it may be necessary to take great care in reducing and finally eliminating the medication.

Patients who have been on MSM, which is derived from DMSO, usually continue on MSM as it is not toxic and can be used when the patient does not want the DMSO breath odor. Those who are using glucosamine sulfate also can continue using it along with the DMSO.

Some patients have said that they feel better if they combine the DMSO with glucosamine sulfate. Others prefer to combine DMSO and MSM. There is no harm in either or both combinations. The individual doctor can observe how his patients perform on the various combinations.

Often patients who have been on prescription medication for many years feel so good that they want to stop all other medication and rely solely on DMSO and other more natural products. This should not be done without medical supervision. If you are a patient who has been on a prescription for a long period of time, you should not stop or reduce the medication on your own no matter how well you feel. It is best to consult the doctor who wrote the original prescription and tell him or her that you feel well and would like to stop the prescription. You may need to stop the medication gradually over a period of days or even months. If this is the case you need professional help to avoid possible severe results.

Any doctor who treats patients who have arthritis should become thoroughly familiar with DMSO. The patient can be treated topically for localized arthritis such as in a finger or in a knee. The patient can be given injections or he can take it by mouth. Various combinations can be given with the doctor making the choice on how best to use the DMSO to best help the patient.

Chapter 5

Athletic Injuries

Athletic injuries have been successfully treated with DMSO for nearly 50 years. When one thinks of athletic injuries, the usual idea is of a sudden injury that may require surgery, setting of a broken bone, or other trauma that requires immediate medical treatment. Actually the more common injury is the one that comes on gradually or after an intense workout or competition. Many times the patient will say there was no single incident, but he thinks there should be an incident that caused the injury.

Actually, any activity or sport that involves constant minor trauma, pounding, or repetitive use of certain muscles, joints, tendons, etc. can lead to a major problem. The extreme effort and fatigue involved in major endurance events, such as marathons, can cause a continual stress that may show up suddenly after many days or months as a painful injury to a knee, hip, or other part of the body.

Repeated small scale trauma to muscle tissue can accumulate and lead to scar tissue and adhesions. When the muscle is worked too hard repeatedly, muscle fiber can be severely damaged or actually destroyed. These injuries can actually make heavy exercise counter-productive in some cases. There is often a narrow margin between beneficial exercise and exercise that does damage. This is especially true of older athletes, such as those in their 60s or 70s.

All the damage listed above can be greatly reduced with DMSO. It is often beneficial to take DMSO just before and shortly after major workouts or competition. As a competitive runner is his 70s, I use compounds containing DMSO every day before I run. Usually it is just applied on the legs. However, a teaspoonful of DMSO is also taken by mouth in juice prior to important races.

What is the reason for using DMSO both before and after competition? The main reason is to reduce inflammation. Also DMSO, as mentioned earlier in this book, is one of the most powerful, if not the absolutely most powerful, free radical scavenger available. Much of the damage in injuries is caused by free radicals after the actual injury. Thus, this damage is prevented or greatly reduced by the proper use of DMSO.

Sam Bell, former track coach at Oregon State University, was one of the first track coaches to use DMSO for the treatment of athletic injuries. In 1963 he had two outstanding runners who were having chronic injuries that were preventing them from training as they should. Morgan Groth, his miler, had a very bad Achilles tendon, and Norm Hoffman, who ran the 880, had a chronic sore hamstring. So coach Bell took both athletes to see Dr. Jacob, and he treated them with DMSO. They were both able to get back into heavy training and both became national champions that year.

Another of Sam Bell's athletes was Darrell Horn, one of the top long jumpers in the country. He had already graduated from Oregon State, and in 1964, he was training for the final trials for the United States Olympic Team. The finals for the long jump were on Saturday and on the Wednesday before the meet he told coach Bell that he was so sore and his hamstring was so discolored that he was not going to jump. Bell flew to Los Angeles and started treating Horn on Thursday morning even though the situation looked hopeless. From the base of his gluteus to three inches below his knee he was black and blue, and he was limping severely. By Saturday afternoon there was no discoloration or soreness. He jumped and missed making the American Olympic Team by three quarters of an inch.

June Connelley, who attracted world-wide attention as a distance runner in 1967 and 1968, is another athlete who was greatly helped with DMSO.

In the late 1960's women were not allowed to officially compete in any Amateur Athletic Union authorized race of over one mile.

This has all changed, and now women routinely run in official races of all distances. However, 45 years ago women were really treated as the weaker sex, and it was feared by some people that the physical demands of running a long race could damage the female body.

Under these conditions, June decided that she could and should be a marathon runner. She was not fast, but she was strong, determined, and had good endurance. There were other problems. She was blind and had been blind since birth. She was also 39 years old. First she needed a coach, so she called this writer and explained the situation. Since she lived in San Francisco, and I lived 400 miles away in Los Angeles, I told her I would find a coach for her in the San Francisco area as I knew several track coaches up there.

It turned out that none of the San Francisco coaches were interested. One of them told me he was not interested in coaching a woman, especially one who was blind. "Besides," he said. "You know it is not legal for her to run over one mile in any race. She's crazy to want to run a marathon. She could have a heart attack. She could also fall down and break a bone. You should really try to talk her out of doing anything this crazy."

Since it was impossible to find her a coach in San Francisco, I finally told her: "If you are crazy enough to try to run a marathon in spite of the difficulties you know you will face, I am crazy enough to be your coach."

She then gained the support of James K. McGee, a sports editor for the San Francisco Examiner, a newspaper in San Francisco. He wrote several excellent sports articles about her running. She was able to get an assistant coach, Don Fletcher, through one of Mr. McGee's articles. A San Francisco doctor also became interested in June's running and promised her free medical treatment to help her running.

It soon became obvious that June had major problems when she trained hard. She had trouble with her Achilles tendon. She had other aches and pains in both legs. These were all treated with

DMSO. Finally she started using DMSO every day on both legs and feet before she ran. This greatly reduced the chance of injury and made her training easier.

June's first race was the Point Reyes marathon, which was located north of San Francisco in December, 1967. When we arrived, the race officials informed us that she could not compete because she was a woman. She was not even to run along the public roads on which the race was to be run.

Tony Stratta, one of the official competitors who ranks among the life time leaders in total miles run in competition in the United States, asked the officials why they did not want her to run. He pointed out that the race was on public roads, and she should be given the chance to see if she could run 26 miles and compete with the men.

She was finally allowed to run unofficially and finished the race along with her coaches who ran the race with her. After he finished the race Mr. Stratta also came back to run the final two miles with June. One of the officials even gave June an orange which caused Mr. McGee to write an article in the San Francisco Examiner asking: "Was the AAU Saved by an Orange?"

The Point Reyes race was just a tune up for the Artesia College Marathon in Artesia, New Mexico, which was held on February 17, 1968. This was one of the largest marathons at that time, and everyone—young, old, male, or female was encouraged to run.

Eight days before the Artesia College Marathon, June was running with her guide dog and stepped into a hole in the sidewalk, twisting her right ankle. For awhile it looked like she would not run at Artesia. Her ankle was sprained and swollen. DMSO was applied to the sprained ankle immediately after the injury. She always carried a small bottle with her when she ran. After the application of the DMSO the ankle felt better. However, she was advised not to run for the next two days. After the two day break, she resumed running lightly until the day of the race.

June ran an excellent race in Artesia. Prior to the race, DMSO was applied to both legs and arms. She also drank one teaspoon of DMSO in cranberry juice approximately one hour prior to the race. June finished third among the women at Artesia. She finished 178th out of 406 runners, male and female, who finished the 26 mile race. Without DMSO it is very doubtful that she would have even run the race. In this instance DMSO really saved the day for us.

What role did June Connelley and DMSO play in later decisions to allow women to officially compete in longer races? We do not know for sure. However, June received very good publicity for her running. She demonstrated that it was possible for a woman who was blind to run a marathon with no damage to her body. It was not long after June's running that the official rules started to change so that now women are allowed to officially run races of all distances.

A large number of professional athletes have used DMSO over the last 40 years. Most don't want to talk about it. Even though DMSO is not a banned substance or listed as a performance enhancing drug, most professional athletes do not like to talk about what they use to reduce down time or to control pain.

Availability to compete is the most important thing to an athlete. If a professional athlete is seriously injured and unable to compete early in his career, the loss of income can be many millions of dollars. There are those who say that we still need double blind studies even for athletic injuries. No athlete wants to be in a control group, and no athlete should be in a control group while others that he has to compete against are using DMSO. All athletes should know about DMSO and feel completely free to use it and discuss it openly for any purpose for which it may be desired.

As this book was being written, there was much concern about brain damage suffered by professional football players who were retired. The brain damage was not the result of a single major injury. The damage came from repeated head trauma during years of hard physical contact while playing football.

Could this brain damage have been reduced by the routine use of DMSO after every football game and also after every practice where there was physical contact where the head was hit or badly shaken? The answer is that most likely the use of DMSO by all players would greatly reduce the chance of major mental problems in the later years of these athletes.

All of the football players could have DMSO applied to their heads after every game and practice. This includes those that have no injury or noticeable damage to the head. Those that showed any sign of possible head injury could also receive the DMSO by injection, thus reducing the possibility of long term damage.

Boxers who are always hit in the head in every boxing match should also receive DMSO treatment after every fight. Various methods of treatment should be tried. DMSO could be applied topically to the head of every boxer, and those who are knocked out or receive head damage could also receive intravenous DMSO immediately after the fight. This treatment would undoubtedly lead to a healthier, happier old age for these athletes.

How about football players, boxers, and other athletes who competed at high levels in contact sports years ago and are now retired from active competition? They should all be using DMSO. The treatment can be as simple as topical application to the head for symptoms of brain damage or to prevent these symptoms. The pateitn could also drink the DMSO in juice or water or the DMSO could be injected. Also the DMSO could be given in combination with other products to further improve the results.

Injuries are to be expected in any extreme athletic competition, but every effort should be made to reduce these injuries and also to allow the athlete to recover from these injuries as rapidly and as completely as possible.

With the proper use of DMSO, these athletes can not only reduce down time, but also reduce the possibility of long term disability.

Chapter 6

Brain Injuries

Severe brain damage, such as that caused by automobile accidents, industrial accidents, falls, or other trauma, can be very difficult to treat by conventional methods. These injuries result in a combination of damage involving nerve injury, free radical formation, edema, decreased blood flow, and a lack of oxygen. The unique properties of DMSO make it the most useful agent known in treating severe head injuries.

DMSO treatment should be started as soon as possible after the injury. However, the statements in some studies and books that treatment must be started within four hours of the injury are not true. There is no definite time limit. Generally the best results are obtained if treatment is started in the first few minutes after the injury. It is a case of the sooner the better and better late than never.

If there is a delay of many hours, there is often permanent damage. Brain tissue is very fragile and can deteriorate rapidly if it is deprived of oxygen. When treatment is delayed certain brain functions can be destroyed permanently or the patient can die.

The usual DMSO treatment for severe head injuries is by the intravenous slow drip method. Up to five grams per kilogram of body weight have been given over a 24 hour period with no toxic side effects. After the first 24 hours, the dosage is usually reduced to two or three grams per kilogram of body weight per day. Often on the first day of treatment the first part of the DMSO dosage is given more rapidly for the first hour of treatment.

Even though the intravenous slow drip method is considered to be the best DMSO treatment for severe head injuries, it does not mean that this should be the first DMSO treatment. Treatment should start as soon as possible. This may mean that the first DMSO treatment should be by an ambulance crew. The treatment could be topical application to the head. Once the patient is in the hospital, the DMSO can then be given by the intravenous route.

When DMSO is infused there is an immediate increase in blood flow to the brain. In head or brain injury much of the permanent damage is caused by a reduction of blood flow into the brain. The reduced blood flow can result in a lack of oxygen and nutrients to brain tissue. If this lasts for a significant period of time, part or all of the brain can be damaged or killed. The final result can be the death of the patient.

Another cause of death or disability in head injuries is an accumulation of blood that compresses the brain. The use of DMSO which results in better blood flow can help the vascular system remove this excess blood from the cranial cavity.

Water can also accumulate in the brain causing pressure on vital parts of the brain. DMSO is the best product available to remove this excess water.

Ten patients with closed head trauma and elevated intracranial pressure were treated with intravenous DMSO in the Division of Neurological Surgery at the University of Dicle in Turkey.[1] The ten patients all had severe closed head injury and had an intracranial pressure monitor installed epidurally through a burr hole shortly after admission. The intracranial pressure of these patients at the time of admission to the hospital ranged from 40 to 127 mm Hg compared to a normal reading of 5 to 13 mm Hg.

DMSO was given by intravenous drip every six hours at a dose of 1.12 grams per kilogram of body weight. Four of the patients received oxygen for the first 24 hours after admission. The dosage of DMSO was reduced by 50 percent when the intracranial pressure dropped to 10 mm Hg and was continued until the intracranial pressure returned to normal or full recovery was obtained.

All patients responded positively to the treatment with an average reduction of intracranial pressure after 24 hours of 28 mm

Hg with DMSO alone and 39 mm Hg with DMSO and oxygen. After six days the average intracranial pressure reduction was 58 mm Hg for DMSO alone and 49 mm Hg with DMSO and oxygen. The lowering of the intracranial pressure was very fast. In most cases the pressure was dropped within the first 30 minutes of treatment. Most patients required treatment for two to 10 days to diminish fluctuation in intracranial pressure.

The reduction in brain swelling following DMSO treatment was confirmed by CT scans. All patients had a neurological assessment six days after the DMSO treatment. Six patients had mild or no problems, two had moderate impairment, and two had severe impairment. Two patients eventually died of their injuries. In a follow up exam three months after discharge seven patients had minimal to no impairment while one patient showed no improvement.

The conclusion was that this study shows that DMSO is effective in reducing intracranial pressure in patients with closed head injury. This study showed improvement in both neurological function and in survival of the patients. There were no adverse side effects, and the DMSO proved safe in relatively high doses over a 10 day period. The researchers recommended more extensive clinical trials in patients with severe injuries.

Jessie Yurick, who now lives in Los Angeles, was 13 years old with an IQ of 165 in August of 1998 when she was thrown off a horse. The horse then landed on her head crushing her safety helmet. Her skull would have been completely crushed without the helmet. She was unconscious for a short time.

On the way to the hospital the paramedics tried to keep her conscious. At this time she was partially conscious and drifting off and on into reality. She was not rational for the next six hours. She then slept for 16 hours. For the next six weeks she was unable to stand by herself. She had severe short term memory problems.

She said her legs felt like they were asleep for four weeks after the accident.

She had severe memory problems that continued for 13 years. She had nerve failure where she would drop things. She was given a variety of medications to help relieve her symptoms, especially her foggy headaches. None of these medications provided much relief and the side effects were often worse than the problem.

Over 13 years later in late 2011 she received her first injection of DMSO. Her mental clarity improved after her first injection. She had more energy and became more positive. As this book is being written her condition is improving rapidly, and she is looking forward to the future.

Based on the proceeding study and other research, it is the opinion of this author that all patients with severe head injuries should receive DMSO treatment. There have been no harmful side effects, and the proper use of DMSO could save the life of many patients with severe head injuries.

[1.] Karaca, M., U.Y. Bilgin, and M. Akar, Dimethyl sulfoxide Lowers ICP After Closed Head Trauma, Division of Neurological Surgery, University of Dicle, Turkey

Chapter 7

Burns

Skin lotions containing DMSO have proven effective in treating burns. Severe burns that cover wide areas of the body can not only be very painful, but these burns can also be fatal. Besides the actual tissue damage, the burn area can become infected.

A Santa Barbara, California cook was carrying a large flat container of hot grease that was nearly boiling. He slipped and fell in the kitchen of the restaurant splattering the grease over a large part of his body. The cook was rushed to the doctor and was found to have second degree burns over much of his body. It was decided to use a lotion containing 50% DMSO and 50% aloe vera on the patient's burns. The first application of lotion was done immediately. Another application was made one hour later. A third application was made three hours after the second. Following this the lotion was applied every eight hours for the next two days.

This man completely recovered from his severe burns. The doctor later said that with any other treatment, recovery would have been slower, and there would possibly have been major complications. One thing he said was certain. There would definitely have been major scarring that would never completely go away. This patient was off work two days. It was estimated that if he had not been given the DMSO treatment, he would have taken over one week to recover sufficiently to return to work.

DMSO lotions have also been used for other types of burns. The application of a DMSO-aloe vera lotion will often prevent the formation of blisters when a person burns a hand on a hot pan. DMSO has also been used to relieve sunburn. Most doctors who treat major burns with DMSO have found the best results come from lotions that combine the DMSO with aloe vera.

Chapter 8

DMSO and Conventional Therapy in the Treatment of Cancer Patients

DMSO has been used successfully in the treatment of cancer for nearly 50 years. There are several properties of DMSO that would tend to make DMSO one of the most important products known to treat cancer. It is a powerful free radical scavenger and detoxifying agent. It can pass through body tissue and individual cells in the body taking other medications with it. DMSO is anti-cancer by itself and much more so when combined with other anti-cancer medications.

Any one of these important properties would indicate that DMSO could be effective in treating cancer. When all of these properties are combined in one product, we have an agent that is one of the most potent anti-cancer medicines known.

Controlled studies have shown DMSO by itself to have a positive effect on cultured leukemia cells. One of the earliest tests reported was conducted by Dr. Charlotte Friend, one of the world's top virologists. In experiments conducted at Mt. Sinai Hospital in New York City, she found that when DMSO was added to the test culture, the cancer cells changed and became like normal cells.

Another study conducted at Nova University in Fort Lauderdale, Florida, combined DMSO with the cancer drug cyclophosphamide, an ester of nitrogen mustard. When given straight the cyclophosphamide lowered the white blood cell count of test rats, and in high doses it killed the rats. When DMSO was given in a low dose in drinking water along with a low dose of cyclophosphamide there was strong anti-cancer activity without the lowered white blood cell count. If the treatment was given early enough, the cancers that were implanted in the rats were killed, and a number of the rats were considered cured.

In tests at other hospitals and medical clinics organisms frequently found in cancer patients and suspected as a cause of some cancers stopped growing when DMSO was added to the culture. Other tests have shown that DMSO, both by itself and in combination with other products, has greatly enhanced the immune system of the body.

A major cancer study that is possibly the most important cancer research ever done was conducted in Chile between 1969 and 1971.[1] A combination of DMSO, amino acids, and cyclophosphamide was used on 65 cancer patients at Military Hospital in Santiago. All patients were classified as incurable, and most had previously been treated with conventional methods. None of the patients had responded favorably to the conventional treatment, and all were expected to die from their cancers.

The toxicity of cyclophosphamide and other chemotherapeutic agents reduces the length of time they can be used. The toxicity of straight chemotherapy also often kills the patient before it kills the cancer. In this study the cyclophosphamide was dissolved in DMSO which greatly reduces its toxicity and at the same time increases its anti-cancer activity.

Oncologists disagree on what dose of cyclophosphamide is most effective in treating cancer. In this study it was decided not to use high and spaced doses of 10-30 mg/kg of body weight by intravenous injection because these doses are dangerous to patients that are very weak, as were most of the patients in this study.

It was decided to give 4-5 mg/kg of body weight either daily or every other day until 3 to 4 grams had been given if the patient did not have any adverse side effects. When the first cycle of treatment was completed, injections were stopped for 12 to 15 days after which another cycle was often administered until another 3 to 4 grams had been given.

Resumption of cycles depended on the remission of the cancer and the general condition of the patient. The total dose of cyclophosphamide given to the patient varied with the average total dose being 6.4 grams. The maximum was 25 grams given to a patient who was treated for over one year. The average total dose of 6.4 grams, which is considered to be low, was sufficient to obtain a remission in a majority of the patients without causing a serious toxic reaction.

The best results were obtained by patients with lymphomas. Twenty two patients were treated with all patients showing subjective remission and 21 of them also having objective remission. Even though all remissions did not last and some patients with remissions did not survive, results were much better than would normally be expected.

Objective or subjective remissions were obtained in 57 of the 65 patients involved in the study. Many of these patients were in extreme pain, and some of these were able to completely discontinue the use of morphine and other pain killers during treatment. Normally the pain caused by the side effects of chemotherapy can be extreme. In this study pain was reduced, not increased, during treatment.

A Los Angeles, California oncologist had a critically ill lymphosarcoma patient that he did not expect to live. The patient and his family were told about the prognosis. The patient then asked his doctor about using DMSO to treat his cancer. The doctor then told the patient that it was possible that he could survive low dose chemotherapy combined with DMSO and that the treatment was legal, but he could not guarantee that the treatment would be successful.

The doctor decided to give this patient intravenous slow drip injections of 4 mg/kg of body weight of cyclophosphamide dissolved in 1 gm/kg of body weight of DMSO. This was given in a normal saline solution four times a week for six weeks.

The patient responded immediately. After one week of treatment he felt better. There were none of the expected side effects of cyclophosphamide, He actually felt better while taking the chemotherapy. At the conclusion of his six week treatment the patient said he felt stronger and healthier than he had felt in years.

This patient also changed his life style. He had smoked over one pack of cigarettes a day his entire adult life and also admitted that he probably drank too much beer. He quit both the cigarettes and beer before treatment started and promised to never use them again. Six years after treatment for terminal lymphosarcoma this man was alive and enjoying good health.

Most, if not all, cancer patients on chemotherapy should receive DMSO as part of their treatment. Side effects of chemotherapy are often extreme and can be fatal. DMSO reduces and sometimes eliminates these toxic side effects, and at the same time it enhances the positive aspects of the chemotherapy. With the proper use of DMSO and chemotherapy cancer survival rates could undoubtedly be greatly increased.

Radiation Therapy for Cancer

The radio protective properties of DMSO have been known for over 40 years. Therefore, it is logical that DMSO should be used as a protective agent when any cancer patient is given radiation. This idea was tested in a study involving cervical cancer patients in Russia and was reported in the Russian radiological journal Meditsinkskaia Radiological. [2]

In this study DMSO was applied topically to 22 cervical cancer patients prior to radiation treatment. The control group consisted of 59 patients who received radiation without the protection of DMSO. The DMSO protected patients did not get the radiation burns normally expected from this treatment. The control group had the normally expected radiation burns along with other toxic reactions.

A Los Angeles lady was suffering from lung cancer. Her doctor decided that she should receive heavy doses of radiation to both lungs. She then told the doctor that she wanted to use DMSO while receiving the radiation. The doctor then told her that she was not to use DMSO or any other product without his approval as it could interfere with the radiation treatment. Actually some studies have shown that DMSO not only provides protection against the toxic effects of the radiation, but it also makes the radiation more effective against the cancer.

At the conclusion of treatment the doctor considered the radiation to be successful. However, this lady suffered severe radiation burns to both lungs. She required oxygen for three months after the conclusion of her radiation treatments. During her worst breathing episodes she was not sure that she would survive.

DMSO therapy that should have been given during her radiation treatments started during the week after the termination of the radiation therapy. This lady received DMSO by injection once a week, drank one teaspoonful twice a day in juice, and applied a lotion containing DMSO to her chest twice a day. Recovery from the radiation burns was rapid. However, based on the Russian study she could probably have avoided these radiation burns entirely by the use of topical DMSO before each radiation treatment.

Another Los Angeles lady was suffering from lung cancer and was referred to a radiologist who decided that this lady should receive a heavy dose of radiation. This radiologist informed the lady that he thought she should receive intense radiation. He also told her that this radiation could severely burn her lungs, and if her lungs were not protected the treatment could cause more harm than good.

This radiologist knew about the Russian study and how the use of DMSO could reduce or eliminate radiation burns. It was mutually agreed that just prior to the radiation DMSO would be applied topically to the patient. The radiation treatment went much better than the patient expected. She had no burns or other adverse side effects from the radiation.

Three years after treatment this patient says that she feels healthy and expects to live many more years. Her doctor agrees and says that it is his opinion that the heavy dose of radiation would have been impossible without DMSO. He thinks the patient would now be dead without the combination treatment.

1. Garrido, J.C., and R.E. Lagos. "Dimethyl Sulfoxide Therapy as Toxicity-Reducing Agent and Potentiator of Cyclophosphamide in the Treatment of Different Types of cancer," *Ann. N.Y. Acad. Sci.*, 245:412-420, 1975.

2. G. M. Zharinov, S.F. Vershinina, and O.I. Drankova "Prevention of Radiation Damage to the Bladder and Rectum Using Local Application of Dimethyl Sulfoxide" Meditsinkskaia Radiologiia 20:16-18 March 1985.

Chapter 9

DMSO and Laetrile in Treating Cancer Patients

DMSO has been used in combination with laetrile in the treatment of cancer since the 1970's. It has been used in a wide variety of ways, including intravenous injections both by the slow drip method and by a push. It has also been administered by intramuscular injections and applied topically directly to the cancer. After the initial treatment, the patient frequently takes laetrile tablets and DMSO by mouth.

The DMSO laetrile combination by the intravenous slow drip method was first officially used by Elmer Thomassen MD in Newport Beach, California in 1977. An artist from New York who had over 30 melanoma tumors on widely scattered parts of his body was flown to California for treatment. This patient was placed on a continuous slow drip using DMSO, laetrile, and vitamin C. In addition DMSO and laetrile were applied topically to his largest tumors.

This patient had an especially large tumor on his shoulder, which is where his cancer originally started. The original cancer had been surgically removed but grew back as other cancer tumors appeared on other parts of his body. This large tumor shrank by nearly 50 percent prior to the death of the patient.

Even though this first patient did not live, the treatment was considered successful. He was in very serious condition and was considered to be terminal with only a few days to live when the DMSO-laetrile treatment was started. He had a major reduction in pain and his condition seemed to improve. The doctor that admitted this patient to the hospital where he died originally had no real hope for the patient, but after one week of treatment, he thought the patient might recover.

The second patient officially treated with the DMSO-laetrile intravenous combination was a lady who was near death with cancer of the tongue along with a staphylococcus infection. She was moved from a hospital to the home of her brother, a medical doctor in Pasadena, California.

This lady was unable to take anything by mouth. DMSO, laetrile, and vitamin C were put in her intravenous solution as soon as she was removed from the hospital. At this time the doctor when told that the treatment should help his sister said "We will know in a couple of days. If she is still alive after two or three days, it will mean that the treatment is successful."

Three days later this lady was eating soft food. Three months later she was leading a normal life and had gained over 20 pounds. She was concerned about her looks and the fact that she was too thin. She remembered nothing about leaving the hospital or what had happened during her worst days. However, by this time this lady was well on her way to complete recovery.

The patient's doctor later said that when the treatment first started he did not think there was any possibility that she would live for one week. He went along with the experiment only because his sister was terminal and he wanted to do everything possible to save her life. He said that it was the most dramatic recovery he had seen in over 30 years of practicing medicine.

This patient continued to use DMSO along with laetrile tablets for several years after her recovery to reduce the chance of the cancer returning. At last contact nearly 10 years after starting treatment this lady was alive and in good health.

Inoperable brain cancer is usually fatal within a short time. In 1979, following brain surgery, a 19 year old lady was told that part of her tumor could not be removed. The surgery was expected to reduce seizures and possibly give additional months of life. However, the surgeon gave no hope for long term survival and said death would probably occur in less than six months.

The family of this young woman decided to have her treated with DMSO and laetrile at the Degenerative Disease Medical Center in Las Vegas, Nevada. DMSO was administered at the rate of one gram per kilogram of body weight (about two ounces) along with six grams of laetrile and 25 grams of vitamin C over a four hour period each day. Treatment was continued for three weeks.

Following the formal treatment at the medical center the patient continued on oral DMSO, laetrile tablets, and vitamins. She was also placed on a healthy diet that emphasized natural and raw foods. Over 20 years later this patient was alive and enjoying relatively good health. Since no brain scan was performed since the original surgery, no one knows what happened to the tumor.

A more recent example of a patient who was treated with the DMSO and laetrile by the slow drip method was a 56 year old man in Los Angeles. He was suffering from prostate cancer. However, he said that the prostate cancer did not concern him that much. His main concern was radiation cystitis which was caused by radiation given to treat his cancer. A surgeon who was treating the patient also said the cystitis was the most immediate problem as the man was bleeding heavily and had recently had several transfusions.

Even though the radiation cystitis was top priority, it was possible to treat both the cystitis and cancer at the same time. This patient received 3 ounces of DMSO along with 25 grams of vitamin C and six grams of laetrile by an intravenous slow drip five days a week for five weeks. He also drank one teaspoonful of DMSO in two ounces of aloe vera juice the same five days a week. On Saturday and Sunday he drank the aloe vera juice and DMSO twice a day.

There was greatly reduced bleeding after three days of treatment. Two weeks later the bleeding completely stopped. At this time the patient said he felt better and stronger than he had felt in months. Three years later this man says he is now feeling the best he has ever felt. He still drinks the DMSO in aloe vera juice every day and says that he intends to stay on this program for the rest of his life.

Many doctors in the United States, Mexico, and other countries have reported success using laetrile and DMSO to treat patients with brain, liver, pancreas, and other cancers that were considered terminal. These doctors explain that the treatment is normally more effective than chemotherapy or radiation. It also has few or no adverse side effects.

Opponents of laetrile, which is also called amygdalin or vitamin B-17, make much of the fact that it contains cyanide which is poisonous. They ignore the fact that many substances that are deadly in sufficient amounts are required by the body. They also ignore the fact that all chemotherapy drugs are toxic and can kill the patient as well as cancer cells. The hope with chemotherapy is that it will kill the cancer before it kills the patient. As pointed out in the previous chapter, the use of DMSO makes the chemotherapy more toxic to the cancer cells and helps protect the normal cells.

How does laetrile work, and why are toxic substances released only at the cancer site? When the laetrile is carried through the body, it is necessary to have a substance to activate the poison. The substance is an enzyme called beta glucuronidase. This enzyme is not found to any dangerous degree anywhere in the body except at the cancer cell where it is always present in great quantities. The result is the laetrile is activated at the cancer cell and nowhere else. The action between the laetrile and beta glucuronidase causes the release of hydrocyanic acid and benzaldehyde, both of which are poisonous by themselves. However, the combination is many times more deadly than either one working by itself.

Normal cells produce another enzyme called rhodanese which cancer cells are unable to produce. Rhodanese neutralizes cyanide and converts it instantly into byproducts that are beneficial to the body. This enzyme is found in every part of the body except the cancer cell.

Beta glucuronidase is found in various concentrations throughout the body, especially in the spleen and liver. However, these organs contain an even greater concentration of rhodanese. Healthy tissue is protected by this excess of rhodanese. The cancer cell which has the greater concentration of beta glucuronidase and is totally lacking in rhodanese is thereby completely defenseless against cyanide.

The diagram on the next page shows how laetrile works to kill the cancer cell, not the cancer patient.

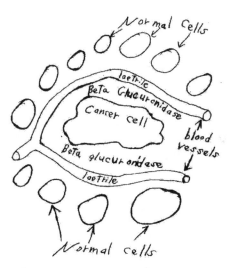

How laeTrile kills Cancer
Not the Cancer PaTienT

Normal Cells

laeTrile
BeTa Glucuronidase
Cancer Cell

blood vessels

BeTa glucuronidase
laeTrile

Normal cells

This drawing shows a cancer cell surrounded by beta glucuronidase. The laeTrile is carried in the blood to the cancer siTe where iT combines with the beTa glucuronidase To form a cyanide compound which kills The cancer cell. The normal cells which conTain much lower levels of beTa glucuronidase produce the enzyme rhodanese which neuTralizes Tha cyanide and converTs iT inTo producTs ThaT are beneficial To The cell.

Chapter 10
Carpal Tunnel Syndrome

Carpal tunnel syndrome is the most commonly reported repetitive strain injury in the workplace. It is caused by compression of the median nerve which results in neuropathy of the nerve. The median nerve is the nerve in the wrist that supplies feelings and movement to parts of the hand. The compression of the median nerve can lead to numbness, tingling, weakness, or muscle damage to the hands and fingers. Long term carpal tunnel syndrome can lead to permanent nerve damage and atrophy of some of the muscles in the hands and fingers.

The conventional treatment has been night splints and cortisone injections. Various anti-inflammatory drugs have also been used. When all else failed, surgery was used to cut the transverse carpal ligament. Surgery has resulted in mixed results. Some patients have found that surgery actually made the condition worse.

Some patients who tried various drugs and even surgery have reported dramatic results with the use of DMSO. Others have reported similar results with MSM (methylsulfonylmethane), a natural substance found in food and the human body which can also be derived from DMSO. Here we will only talk about DMSO, even though MSM has also proven helpful.

DMSO can provide a number of benefits to the person with carpal tunnel syndrome. First DMSO is an anti-inflammatory without any of the harmful side effects of some commonly used anti-inflammatory drugs. This is very important because inflammation in the wrist can cause compression on the median nerve. DMSO can also help by improving circulation in the area and reducing pain.

One Los Angeles man with carpal tunnel syndrome was especially troubled with one of his thumbs. He was diagnosed with "trigger thumb" where his thumb would be so stiff in one position that he could not move it. He had previously had hand surgery. He said the surgery made the condition worse.

This man was finally treated with topical DMSO. The DMSO was applied twice a day to his thumb, all fingers, his hand and his arm up to his elbow. Relief was immediate. He felt better after the first application, and he had no problem at all with the thumb after two weeks. He considered himself to be cured.

Chapter 11

Cirrhosis of the Liver

Cirrhosis of the liver can result in a very unpleasant death for the patient. A number of patients near the downtown area of Los Angeles who were heavy users of alcohol, had poor diets, and lived mostly on the streets were ill, vomiting, and had other digestive symptoms. A group of these patients were found to be suffering from cirrhosis of the liver. These patients were considered terminal, but they did want to live. First they were told that they could possibly be helped with an experimental program using DMSO. They were told that if it was discovered that they were drinking any beer, wine, or other alcoholic beverage, they would be dropped from the program.

These patients were given one teaspoonful of DMSO in one ounce of aloe vera juice two times a day for a period of six months. Twelve patients started the program, and eight continued for the full six months. These eight patients all experienced greatly improved health, greatly reduced vomiting, and improved liver function tests. Prior to treatment all eight of these patients were expected to be dead within one year. However, after one year all were alive and functioning better than when they had first started the study.

This study does not mean that a person who has severe liver damage can simply use DMSO and continue to abuse his body with alcohol or other products. The patient must also stop the process that is damaging to the body. DMSO does help to heal the body naturally.

Chapter 12

Diabetes

Patients with both Type 1 and Type 2 diabetes have reported good results using DMSO as part of their treatment. This does not mean the patient can stop using insulin. However, some patients have been able to reduce the use of insulin through daily use of DMSO. No patient should change his insulin without the approval of his doctor.

DMSO has shown great potential in treating diabetic neuropathy. This is often a major problem in older people who have suffered from diabetes for many years. A good example of this is a Los Angeles area man who had diabetes all his life. By the time he was 64 years old he was having trouble walking. He had poor circulation and suffered from severe neuropathy of the lower legs and both feet. He said he could not even feel the ground when he walked. This man was treated with topical DMSO twice a day on both feet and legs. He also drank one teaspoon of DMSO in juice every evening after dinner. He was instructed to be more careful following his diabetic diet. Even though he did not like it, he was also given an exercise program. He was told that if he did not do everything correctly, he would probably completely lose his ability to walk.

Within a few weeks the feeling started to return to his feet. He could feel when his feet hit the ground. This man will probably remain on insulin for the rest of his life, but with the proper use of DMSO, diet, and exercise, he is able to enjoy a happier, more active life.

Another severe diabetic case involved a Ventura, California engineer with circulation problems in his feet. He was told that two toes should be surgically removed. There was no chance to save the toes and any delay could result in loss of at least part of the foot according to the surgeon. This engineer was totally opposed to amputation. DMSO was applied topically to all the toes, both feet and both legs. The toes that were scheduled to be amputated gradually improved so no surgery was done.

DMSO improves the blood supply by dilating the small blood vessels thereby increasing circulation to the extremities. DMSO should be part of the normal medical treatment of every diabetic. The treatment should not wait until there is a major circulation problem where amputation is considered. Prevention of the problem should be the goal. It is probable that most diabetic related amputations could be prevented with routine DMSO treatment for all diabetics.

Chapter 13

Digestive Problems

Digestive disorders of various types can be very difficult to treat and even more difficult to diagnose. A good example involved an eight year old girl in Los Angeles who vomited daily after breakfast. She was a recent immigrant to the United States and was staying with an aunt. She was taken to a doctor who said that the girl was suffering from internal bleeding. He referred the girl to a specialist who found that she had a partial blockage caused by a very bad fungus infection.

The specialist thought that the infected part of the intestinal tract would probably have to be removed by surgery. Some conventional anti fungus medications were tried without success. As a last result before surgery, it was decided to try DMSO. She was given ½ a teaspoon full of DMSO in one ounce of aloe vera diluted with two ounces of water after breakfast and dinner. The vomiting stopped after three days. The treatment was discontinued. A week later, the symptoms returned. After this, the treatment was resumed and continued for two weeks after all the symptoms had disappeared. Fifteen years later the problem had not returned.

This is an example of an open minded doctor who wanted to avoid surgery on a child. His decision to try DMSO before resorting to surgery saved the girl from major intestinal surgery that could have caused her trouble for the rest of her life.

Many DMSO studies have been conducted by Dr. Aws Salim, regarded by many as the top researcher in treating free radical damage. Several studies have been conducted under his direction to see if gastric problems could be reduced by the proper use of free radical scavengers.

One study investigated whether stress induced mucosal injury in patients with pelvic fractures and hypovolemic shock could be reduced by the use of DMSO or allopurinol.[1] This study included 177 patients with 57 receiving DMSO, 62 receiving allopurinol, and 58 serving as controls. Patients in both the DMSO and allopurinol groups showed positive results over those in the control group.

During the first three days after hospitalization 13 patients in the control group developed stress induced gastric mucosal injury while only two patients in each of the DMSO and allopurinol group developed this injury. Eight patients in the control group and one patient in the allopurinol group deteriorated so that emergency surgery was required. Three patients in the control group died shortly after surgery while all patients in the DMSO and allopurinol groups survived.

The conclusion of this study was that free radicals are implicated in stress induced gastric mucosal injury and that removing the free radicals provides protection and reduces the chance of death from this injury.

Another study by Dr. Salim was conducted to determine whether or not free radicals are involved in the recurrence of duodenal ulcers. This study involved 302 patients with ulcers that had healed. All patients were smokers and social drinkers. These patients were divided randomly into four groups to receive either DMSO, allopurinol, cimetidine, or to serve as a placebo for a one year period.

The relapse rate where the ulcer returned during the year was placebo 65%, cimetidine 30%, DMSO 13% and allopurinol 12%. While the conventional treatment of cimetidine was much more effective than the placebo this study showed that the free radical scavengers DMSO and allopurinol provided the best protection against the return of duodenal ulcers.

Five ulcer patients in New York City had suffered from duodenal ulcers off and on for over 10 years. All were social drinkers, and it was suspected that the drinking was heavier than admitted in at least two of the patients. These patients were all treated with one teaspoonful of DMSO in two ounces of aloe vera juice three times a day until the ulcer was shown endoscopically to have healed. During the next year the patients were advised to take one teaspoonful of DMSO in two ounces of aloe vera juice every evening.

These patients were all examined monthly during the one year test period. All reported that they had no ulcer symptoms. Their health was better than expected, and their work attendance was excellent. Three of the patients did not miss any work days because of illness during the test period. Breath odor was controlled with chlorophyll and breath mints.

Ulcers and acute gastric mucosal injury can not only provide the patient with much pain, they can also result in the death of the patient unless properly treated. DMSO treatment is easy for the doctor and the patient and should probably be tried on every ulcer patient.

An interesting case where the patient was originally misdiagnosed involved a 55 year old woman with severe digestive problems. She was suffering from internal bleeding, shortness of breath, overall weakness, and fainting spells that were becoming increasingly worse. She finally consulted with a top specialist at a well known medical center in California. This doctor diagnosed her with angiodysplasia, an age related deterioration of the gastro-intestinal tract.

By then her hemoglobin was down to 5.0 and she required an immediate blood transfusion. After that the prescribed treatment consisted of intravenous iron injections. When the iron injections failed to stabilize her hemoglobin, regular blood transfusions were given every few months in addition to the intravenous iron. This continued over a period of three years. This treatment created other complications, and by late 2005 as her condition grew worse she was considered terminal. She was receiving blood transfusions every month by this time, but the hematologist that was treating her said she had the potential for sudden massive bleeding at any time. While he did not know when this would occur the hematologist said it would probably happen within the next six months with a fatal result.

At this time her daughter did some investigating on her own and found someone else to also treat her mother. It was discovered that she did not have angiodysplasia. She did have deterioration of the gastric-intestinal tract, but it was not age related.

This lady had suffered from severe chronic headaches since she was a girl. She began self-medication with aspirin to control the pain in her head. Finally she started using aspirin every day. Over time she found that aspirin taken with Coca Cola seemed to make her feel even better. She was then informed that her actual problem was not age related, but that she had severely damaged her gastro-intestinal tract from many years of daily aspirin and Coca Cola.

After the correct diagnosis was made, she was put on DMSO and other products in an attempt to save her life. She was given injections of DMSO, B-12, and other medications twice a week. She was told that she had to cut her dependency on aspirin and Coca Cola. She was told to use a DMSO compound topically for her headaches. She was also told that since she did not completely stop the aspirin and Coca Cola she should at least use one teaspoonful of DMSO in two ounces of aloe vera juice before taking the Coca Cola and aspirin.

Six years later, this lady is still alive. She has not received a blood transfusion since her DMSO treatment started. She has now completely stopped the aspirin and Coca Cola. She has not completely stopped the bleeding, and she has some damage that will never be completely healed. However, she is now no longer in danger of dying from this problem in the near future.

There are some basic lessons to be learned from the problem of the previous lady. The first thing any medical professional should realize is that the best specialist can make a major mistake in diagnosing a patient. It is always important to get as much information as possible about the patient. Especially with problems anywhere in the digestive system, the doctor should ask about diet, medications, and other products the patient may be taking. These have to be specific questions. Often the patient will not give information that is really important because it is not considered to have anything to do with the problem.

The doctor needs to be extremely observant. In the preceding case the patient told her hematologist that she took a small amount of aspirin, and she actually carried with her to her doctor's appointment an open bottle of Coca Cola from which she had been drinking. He asked no questions of the patient and just assumed that her problem was age related when it was actually caused by products that she had taken in to her body.

Years ago this author briefly worked for Elmer Thomassen, a Newport Beach, California surgeon. One of his employees gave a new patient a very detailed questionnaire that the doctor wanted filled out before he saw the patient. This patient told the doctor that most of the questions did not really apply in her case. Dr. Thomassen replied "I am not smart enough to know what is important until I see your answers. Then I may know what answers are important."

The doctor can sometimes tell what is wrong with the patient with exams, blood tests, etc., but often the cause is not so obvious. This writer does not know personally of any cases where a patient has actually died of age related deterioration of the gastro-intestinal tract. He does know of cases where a patient has died because of combining aspirin and Coca Cola or using other products that have resulted in damage, severe bleeding, and death.

DMSO can greatly reduce the damage to the digestive system especially when it is combined with other products such as aloe vera. However, it is often not the final answer. You always need to find the true cause or causes of the patient's problem. The cause then needs to be removed or at the very least reduced as much as possible

[1.] Salim, A. S. Protection Against Stress Induced Gastric Mucosal Injury by Free Radical Scavengers, Intensive Care Med 1991:17(8): 455-460.

Chapter 14

Ear & Hearing Problems

Ear problems affect a large part of the population. Many small children have ear infections nearly every year. This is often treated by puncturing the eardrum to release pus and relieve pressure. This operation is very painful. In many cases DMSO in combination with an anesthetic makes it possible to puncture the eardrum without the normal severe pain. In other cases the patients with middle or inner ear infection may be treated with DMSO combined with an antibiotic without puncturing the eardrum.

One family in Los Angeles had six children, all of whom had ear infections as babies and young children. Even though the weather was never really cold, these children would get their ear infections in the winter. One winter the three youngest children aged seven, eight, and nine all had ear infections. They complained of pain and also had some hearing problems. This time the children were treated with DMSO. An eye dropper was used to place two drops of 50% DMSO in each ear. A 90% solution was also applied to the head and neck area near the ears. There was immediate relief. The mother of the children was advised to continue the treatment at home with drops of DMSO in the ears twice a day and to have the drops available to treat the ears of her children at the first sign of trouble. The children remained infection free for the rest of the winter.

The childrens' doctor advised their mother to treat the children with the DMSO ear drops at least once a week during the following winter. This was done, and none of the children had any more ear trouble. Of course there is no proof that the children would have had an infection without the drops. However, it is probable that at least one of them would have had an ear infection without the treatment.

Tinnitus

Tinnitus, which is a condition in which the patient suffers from a variety of ear noises, is a frequent cause of visits to the ear, nose, and throat specialist. The most common noise is a hissing, buzzing, or ringing sound. However, there can be great variety in the noise. In some patients it may even be music. The problem may be constant or occasional and is often accompanied by at least a partial hearing loss. If the noise is continuous and intense, it can severely affect both the physical and mental health of the patient.

Prior to the use of DMSO there was very little that could be done to relieve the symptoms of tinnitus. Surgery was tried in some cases. Other times doctors thought the problem might be an infection and tried various antibiotics without success. In some cases it was even suggested that the patient might have mental problems. There was no real noise, but the patient could definitely hear the buzzing, hissing or even music when there was none present.

A study conducted in Chile and presented at the New York Academy of Sciences 1975 Conference on DMSO by Aristedes Zuniga Caro showed excellent results in treating tinnitus with DMSO.[1] Fifteen patients who had suffered from tinnitus for a minimum of six months were included in the study. None of the patients had adapted to the noise.

The patients were treated for one month with a DMSO spray combined with anti-inflammatory and vasodilatory drugs applied in the ear canal every four days for one month. The patients also received an intramuscular injection of DMSO and the other medications every day.

All patients had at least some relief. Nine completely recovered from the tinnitus, and no symptoms returned during the following year. Four who had continuous symptoms prior to treatment had only occasional symptoms after treatment. Two patients had a continuation of the noises but a lower intensity.

Other symptoms also improved. Prior to treatment 11 patients suffered from headaches. Seven of these were completely cured, and three others had less severe symptoms. All patients also had insomnia. This completely stopped in eight patients, and the others all had some benefit.

It was also noted that the ear temperature rose from 36.8 C before treatment to 37.9 C after the treatment. This would indicate an improvement of the blood flow in the inner ear which may be one reason for the improvement of all the symptoms. The average normal temperature in 10 adults without ear problems was 38.1 C.

The exact DMSO treatment for tinnitus has varied based on the desires of both the doctor and the patient. The treatments in many cases were very simple, and the results were very positive.

A number of tinnitus patients were treated with DMSO at a New York City clinic. The treatment consisted of ear drops of 40 percent DMSO deposited in the ear each day. Also, a lotion containing 90 percent DMSO combined with capsicum and aloe vera was applied around each ear twice a day. The ear noises in most cases were reduced almost immediately. Usually the patient was considered cured within one month. The symptoms did not normally come back. If they did, the DMSO treatment was redone, and relief was normally more rapid than during the first treatment.

This clinic treated patients for a variety of problems. Many times patients had other complaints and did not even mention any ear problems. They would be treated for the other problem, and the treatment included DMSO. Later they would mention the noise in their ears and say that it had improved. This often happened even when there was no treatment to the ears. In these cases the ears were then usually treated, and complete relief was obtained.

[1.] Aristides Zuniga Caro "Dimethyl Sulfoxide Therapy in Subjective Tinnitus of Unknown Origin" Annals of the New York Academy of Sciences Volume 243 pgs. 468-474

Chapter 15

Emergency Medicine

DMSO has proven to be so effective in treating such a wide variety of conditions and injuries with no harmful side effects that one would expect it to be used in all emergency rooms. It would also be logical for all who are trained in first aid to receive instruction on the use of DMSO.

It has been suggested that all ambulances and paramedical units should carry DMSO. Over 30 years ago Bruce Halstead, M.D., a Southern Californian doctor, stated "Hopefully DMSO will soon be available in all emergency rooms and ambulances and all emergency medical personnel will be properly trained in the use of DMSO." At the time this book was being written DMSO was still not widely available in most emergency rooms.

There have been no logical arguments presented against the use of DMSO under emergency procedures. There are certain properties of DMSO that make it a highly desirable agent in treating victims of major accidents or sudden serious illnesses such as strokes or heart attacks. DMSO reduces edema, is anti-inflammatory, increases oxygen supply and as a free radical scavenger helps protect the cells from mechanical damage.

Over 30 years ago there was an industrial medicine clinic in Los Angeles that regularly used DMSO on most patients that came to the clinic. The majority of the patients were injured on their jobs and were seen shortly after the injury. Many of the patients were seen within minutes of their injuries. Often these patients were treated with DMSO before the patient was fully evaluated. This was done to prevent the damage from the injury from progressing needlessly while the patient was being examined. The doctors at this clinic knew DMSO could help a wide variety of problems and even if it was not beneficial in every case there was very little chance of doing any damage to the patient. Usually the first DMSO treatment at this clinic was topical applied to the area of injury.

Another example involved an uninformed emergency room doctor in the San Gabriel Valley east of Los Angeles. A lady had a major stroke and was taken by ambulance at night to the hospital. Her family wanted her to be treated with DMSO. The emergency room doctor said that he would not allow DMSO because he had never heard of it, and the patient was going to die anyway. A nurse who was treating the patient agreed with the family and helped with the DMSO. In the morning a neurosurgeon took charge of the patient and ordered DMSO be added to her intravenous injection. He said he did not expect it to be beneficial in this case because of the severe damage, but that he would want it done if the patient were his wife or mother.

United States congressional representative Gabrielle Giffords was shot in the head and seriously injured while this book was being written. A number of people asked if she should be treated with DMSO. The answer is she should have definitely been treated with DMSO. The treatment would have improved her condition. No one knows for sure how much it would have benefited her, but my guess is that there would have been dramatic improvement. Even now when you are reading this, even if it is years later, she would probably receive some benefit from DMSO.

A good example where DMSO was used immediately is a Los Angeles nurse who was hit by a car while crossing the street. She was knocked down, but no bones were broken. She was in pain from multiple injuries and said that she was sure that she would not be able to walk the next day. She expected extreme stiffness with delayed adverse reactions from the accident.

DMSO was applied topically to much of the body of this nurse less than 10 minutes after the accident. She also drank one teaspoonful of DMSO in a small glass of juice. Two hours later

DMSO was again applied topically. Even though she was familiar with DMSO, she was surprised at how well she felt. By this time she had very little pain from the accident.

The next morning this patient was feeling much better and had no stiffness. She made the comment that the DMSO really helped. She also said that she did not think the accident was as bad as originally thought. She really expected to be suffering major disability from the accident for a week or more.

Hopefully in the near future DMSO will be prescribed in most emergency medical situations. Especially topical application is so simple and safe that nearly anyone can be trained to use it safely and effectively.

Chapter 16

Eye Problems

Even though DMSO had been temporarily banned and all research was stopped in the 1960s because of possible toxicity to the eyes of dogs and rabbits, DMSO has since not only been proven to be non-toxic to the eyes of humans, it is used directly in the eye to reverse conditions that could otherwise lead to blindness.

Some of the most dramatic vision improvement with the use of DMSO has occurred in the treatment of retinitis pigmentosa. Retinitis pigmentosa is a leading cause of blindness. The DMSO treatment is simple and effective.

One of the first doctors to use DMSO in the eyes was Doctor Robert Hill of Longview, Washington. His early studies were reported in the January 1975 annals of the New York Academy of Science.[1] One early patient with retinitis pigmentosa could see only hand motion with his right eye and had 20/200 vision in his left eye. Treatment, which consisted of 50% DMSO by eyecup twice daily, was started on February 10, 1972. Five days later the patient's vision improved to 20/70 in the left eye and could count fingers at five feet with his right eye. Three months later his vision was 20/50 in the left eye. A later visual test in 1974 found his vision still 20/50 in his left eye and he could count fingers at six feet with his right eye.

A later study by Dr. Hill involved 50 patients with deterioration caused by either retinitis pigmentosa or macular degeneration. Of the 50 DMSO treated patients, 22 had improved visual acuity, nine had improved visual fields and five improved in dark adaption. Only two patients out of the 50 continued to get worse. The remaining patients had no noticeable changes in vision. Without the treatment it is probable that all 50 patients would have continued to regress.

Later patient treatments have shown positive results in not only retinal problems, but other eye disorders as well. In some cases the treating physician does not know for sure what is causing an eye problem. In these cases treatment with DMSO is usually indicated. There have been many times that a patient is treated with DMSO for arthritis or an injury, and the eyes also get better.

Many doctors have reported positive results with a 40% DMSO solution applied to the eye with an eye dropper. When this treatment is done usually one drop is applied in each eye once a day. This can be done for all problems involving vision or pain in the eyes. When the DMSO is applied there is normally a stinging sensation in the eye for 30 or 40 seconds. This is no cause for worry. Normally after the very brief stinging the eyes will feel better than before the treatment.

DMSO has also been used successfully to treat vision problems of the elderly. One Los Angeles area doctor reported that several patients were able to more easily read fine print after only one week of using 40% DMSO eye drops.

One 90 year old man was unable to read. He was highly educated and owned his own successful business that he had sold 15 years before when he was 75. He had a large collection of books that he had planned to read during his retirement years. However, by the time he reached 90 he had macular degeneration and other eye problems that made it impossible to read. His wife read some items to him, but for his books he hired outside readers. He was treated daily with 40% DMSO eye drops. One drop was placed in each eye every day. He also drank one teaspoon of DMSO daily in orange juice. His vision improved during the first week of treatment. One month after starting treatment this man was able to resume reading the books in his collection. He also said he could think more clearly and his whole body felt better.

A 78 year old Los Angeles man suffered from a variety of eye problems and was having trouble walking and working around his house. He was told by his doctor that he should get used to having vision problems and that his eyes would gradually get worse until he was completely blind. He was also told there was nerve deterioration and other problems that could not be treated. The doctor said he should accept the inevitable and not waste his time and money on any unproven treatment.

This man decided he would not take "no treatment" for an answer. He visited another doctor and showed him an article about using DMSO to treat various eye problems. The new doctor told him that he considered the treatment to be unproven but said it was worth trying because the treatment was not dangerous. One drop of 40% DMSO was applied in each eye by the doctor. The patient was also advised to take one teaspoonful of DMSO in a small glass of juice each day. The wife of this patient later applied the eye drops in each of his eyes each day. The doctor examined the eyes every two weeks. Vision that was 20/200 improved to 20/100 in two weeks. A month later the patient's vision was 20/70. His vision later improved to 20/50 with glasses. This patient has continued his treatment at home for several years. He now sees his doctor every three months for an examination and evaluation. He is considered to be in excellent health for a man in his 80s.

This writer has used DMSO eye drops with 40% DMSO in his own eyes when the eyes have felt tired. There has always been immediate relief. After the initial stinging the eyes always feel fresh with no pain.

[1.] Hill, Robert V. "Dimethyl Sulfoxide in the Treatment of Retinal Disease" Annals of the New York Academy of Sciences, Volume 243, pgs. 485-493

Chapter 17

Fibromyalgia

Fibromyalgia is a relatively common rheumatic disease that affects women much more often than men. The incidence increases with age and is most common in women over 50. Unlike arthritis, fibromyalgia attacks the muscles, tendons, and ligaments.

It is a difficult ailment to diagnose because many other problems have similar symptoms. The diagnosis of this problem generally requires widespread pain that lasts for more than three months and affects all four quadrants of the body—both sides and above and below the waist. There is also painful response to pressure.

Some patients have bowel and bladder problems. Others have difficulty in swallowing. It is frequently associated with psychiatric conditions such as anxiety and depression. Symptoms vary widely from patient to patient, and some of the symptoms are completely lacking in some patients. The cause of fibromyalgia is unknown. One theory is that these patients have a lower threshold of pain because of increased sensitivity to pain signals.

Conventional treatment consisting of painkillers, cortisone, and antidepressants has not had good results. Much better results have often been obtained using DMSO and MSM.

A 75 year old Los Angeles lady had been diagnosed with fibromyalgia three years earlier. At first she had been told that there was nothing wrong with her and that it was all in her head. However, she knew that she had a major problem. She could hardly walk because of the severe pain. She was referred to a psychiatrist who found her mentally sound, and he suggested that she might have fibromyalgia. This was later confirmed by another doctor. She was prescribed painkillers and cortisone, but the side effects were nearly as bad as the original problem.

It was finally suggested that she receive DMSO by a slow drip over a period of three hours. She felt better after the first treatment and continued taking three treatments a week for 10 weeks. On her off days she drank one teaspoonful of DMSO in juice. After the 10 week treatment she took DMSO in juice every day for about one year. After this she replaced the DMSO with 10 grams of MSM per day. Since the original treatment with DMSO, this lady has been able to enjoy a life that is mostly free of pain.

Chapter 18

Fungus Infections

DMSO has proven very effective in the treatment of fungus infections and other infections of the skin. It has been used successfully to treat problems ranging from athletes foot and jungle rot to acne.

Jungle rot is a serious infection that is found in hot moist areas. Many veterans became infected with jungle rot in the South Pacific during the Second World War. Others became infected in Vietnam. Usually those that became infected had not been able to have good foot hygiene. Their feet became wet in the hot jungle and they were unable to change their socks and shoes for many days. This provided a perfect environment for any fungus, especially jungle rot. Once a patient contracts jungle rot, it is very difficult to treat.

Dr. Robert Entin of Los Angeles was one of many veterans of the Second World War who became infected with jungle rot in the South Pacific. He said that he had spent thousands of dollars of his own money in addition to the government money through the Veterans' Administration in an attempt to obtain relief. Finally he used a skin lotion containing DMSO and aloe vera. He obtained immediate relief. The lotion did not completely cure the infection. It was still in his system and did come back later. However, the lotion provided much more relief than any other medication that he had used.

The lotion was later used by a Veterans' Administration doctor in Los Angeles to treat a number of veterans. The results in each case were excellent. There was immediate relief. However, in every case there were later infections because the fungus was not completely killed. The doctor who treated these patients later said that he considered the DMSO lotion to be the best treatment for jungle rot and that he thought it should be used on every veteran with any type of fungus infection.

In the preceding examples the jungle rot was controlled, but not completely cured using a DMSO lotion. The infections did come back during hot summer weather unless treatment was continued.

Athlete's foot is another fungus infection that responds well to DMSO treatment. The DMSO has been used in concentrations ranging from 50% to 90% DMSO. In some cases other products such as capsicum pepper and aloe vera are mixed with the DMSO. Athlete's foot is often a chronic condition that recurs during the summer, especially if the person wears enclosed shoes that do not allow for heat and moisture to be dispersed. The DMSO will sometimes completely cure this fungus infection. However, it is also important to allow the shoes to thoroughly dry and air out to kill any fungus spores in the shoes.

Fungus under the finger nails and toe nails can also be treated with the topical application of DMSO. Usually the DMSO is applied both on the nail and on the finger or toe in the area of the infection. These are usually treated twice a day until the infection is gone.

Foot odor that is not caused by infection can be an annoying and smelly problem. This smell is not necessarily due to poor foot hygiene. Clean dry socks and clean dry feet can reduce this problem, but often not completely eliminate it. DMSO applied lightly to both feet usually stops foot odor and eliminates excess moisture on the feet. Temporary relief is often obtained with one application of DMSO. Long term relief usually requires repeated application. Generally the longer the DMSO is applied, the longer the odor stays away after treatment is discontinued.

Chapter 19

Hair and Scalp Problems

DMSO has been used to stimulate hair growth for at least 40 years. Patients that have recently lost hair usually have the best results. A man who has been bald for many years is very unlikely to experience great improvement or a full head of hair from the use of DMSO or any other product. When hair growth occurs, the last areas that lost hair are the first to grow new hair.

The hair growth has also been observed in animals treated with DMSO. Cats that had suffered severe hair loss in a few instances had the hair grow back completely when treated with a topical lotion containing DMSO. Other cats, which had not lost hair, had thicker hair on areas treated with DMSO.

Both men and women who had lost hair during cancer chemotherapy grew hair back much more rapidly than expected when a DMSO lotion was applied to their heads. The oncologist that reported these results did not expect very rapid hair regrowth. He had these patients experiment with the treatment because he knew the DMSO would not harm the patient, and the patients were anxious to have hair.

Why does DMSO stimulate hair growth? The primary reason is that DMSO being an excellent vasodilator, dilates the small capillaries in the scalp. There is then increased blood supply to the roots of the hair. Needed nutrients are then brought to the hair follicles allowing the growth of hair to begin again. With normal male pattern baldness the hair growth is usually slow but many patients have reported positive results.

This author has used a DMSO lotion on his hair for over 20 years with the goal of keeping a full head of hair. At the age of 75 he still has his normal brown hair. There is no way to prove that this is the result of using DMSO, but it is probable that if DMSO were not used there would be some hair loss and also loss of hair color.

An 80 year old man in Oklahoma was having seepage of a sticky substance from his scalp. He sought medical help and was then referred to a specialist. The specialist recommended a procedure where this patient would be scalped. The specialist said the patient had an infection under his scalp and the best way to treat the infection was to surgically remove part of the scalp to expose the infected area. The patient rejected this procedure as too extreme. Finally a DMSO lotion was applied to his head. Six months later, there was no infection, and the patient had a healthy scalp.

Chapter 20
Headache

Headaches of various types affect most people at some point in their lives. In fact nearly half of the population has at least one headache a month. Most headaches are at least partially caused by muscle spasms in the neck and changes in blood vessels going into the head. Emotional stress and the way the body reacts to it is often an underlying cause.

Aspirin is frequently the first treatment used by most headache sufferers. The results may vary, but especially with migraine headaches, the pain reduction is often minimal.

DMSO has been used to treat headaches for over 40 years. The results have generally been good, and there is the lack of side effects found with many of the conventional pain medication.

Migraine headaches that have developed to full strength do not seem to respond well to any treatment. However, it has been observed that if a migraine headache is treated in the early stages, the condition can be reversed with DMSO. This has happened with a number of patients. It is important that the patient receive the DMSO treatment early in the pain process.

The usual DMSO treatment for headache is topical application to the head, neck, or both. The topical application can also be enhanced by injecting the DMSO or having the patient drink it in juice or water.

One interesting headache case was a young woman in Newport Beach, California. She was having frequent headaches that had been getting worse over a period of months. An x-ray examination of her head revealed a thin film of unknown origin. It was decided to start topical and oral DMSO treatment on the lady. DMSO was applied on the total head except for the face. She was also given one teaspoon of

DMSO in four ounces of water to drink. She was then told to do the same treatment at home every day until her next appointment.

Ten days later this lady returned to the clinic and was asked if she still had headaches. She said yes, and the headaches had gotten worse. She had previously said that the treatment had helped her, and she felt better. Finally she admitted what she had done. Since she felt better with the small dose of DMSO, she decided to increase the dosage. She said she drank four ounces of DMSO the morning after her original appointment. Then she added that it was taken with one quart of water. Instead of following her doctor's instructions, she just figured that if a little is good a lot is a lot better.

This is just one more example of a patient who did not follow instructions. She was told that with many drugs an extreme overdose can be fatal. Luckily for this lady DMSO is very safe even at higher than recommended dosages. Whenever a patient has an unexpected side effect it can be beneficial to ask the patient the dosage taken and how the medication was used. If the patient is asked if a drug was used as prescribed by the doctor the usual answer is yes. However, if instead the patient is asked how the product was used and how much was used, correct information is more likely to be provided to the doctor.

In this particular case after she followed the prescription given by her doctor, the headaches of the lady diminished and she was completely free of her headaches six months later. During the six month period she drank only one teaspoon of DMSO along with the topical application. Since she did not return to the clinic in the years following the six months of treatment, it is assumed that she did not have any problem in the following years.

Chapter 21

Infections

DMSO has proven valuable both by itself and in combination with antibiotics and other products in the treatment of a wide variety of infections.

A 43 year old Los Angeles man in the moving business had a heavy box dropped on his right foot causing a severe crushing injury. The injury would not heal and became infected. Various antibiotics were tried, but the infection would not heal and started to spread. The possibility of amputation was discussed. Finally DMSO was given intravenously in combination with the antibiotics. There was immediate improvement. Two weeks later this patient was walking on the infected foot. One month later this patient was back at work, and he now has no problem with the foot.

Osteomyelitis is a serious and difficult to treat infection of the bone. Often amputation is required to save the life of the patient if an extremity is involved. Other times, especially when amputation is not an option, the infection will be fatal. The first treatment is nearly always strong antibiotic treatment. This is often not successful, especially if the patient did not seek medical help early in the infection process.

A 36 year old Santa Monica, California man stepped on a large nail that penetrated deep into his foot. He treated the wound himself with the help of his wife. The injury seemed to heal, and this man forgot about the injury even though he still had some pain. Finally after two months he decided to seek medical help for the pain in the foot. No obvious injury was present, and he neglected to tell the doctor about the nail. Pain killers were prescribed and the patient seemed to improve.

Three months later this patient returned to the doctor. The pain was worse, and he had trouble walking. An examination showed damage to the bone. The patient was then questioned about any injury to the foot. Finally he mentioned the nail, but only after he was asked if he had ever stepped on a nail. He said yes he had, and it was close to the area of his pain. However, that injury was completely healed so he did not think the pain was caused by the injury. This man had osteomyelitis, an infection of the bone marrow.

Strong antibiotics were given with only slight temporary improvement. The possibility of amputation was discussed. As a last resort, DMSO was combined with the antibiotics. There was immediate improvement. Within less than one month all signs of the infection were gone, and there has been no problem with the foot since the DMSO treatment.

Unfortunately there has been a lack of good recognized studies of DMSO combined with various antibiotics in the treatment of infection. Doctors who use DMSO in their medical practice frequently use DMSO along with antibiotics to treat infections. However, the treatment and the results of the treatment are usually not written up or publicized.

Based on my observation and experience with various infections, this writer, who is not a medical doctor and has never claimed to be one, believes that all major infections should be treated with a combination of DMSO and antibiotics. This is especially true if the infections do not respond to conventional antibiotic treatment.

A 90 year old Los Angeles man was suffering from a severe bladder infection. Twenty five years earlier he had prostate surgery which caused severe urinary problems. Prior to his infection this man had been on diapers for many years due to his inability to control his urine. He also had other medical problems which made it difficult for him to walk even using a walker.

This patient was admitted to the hospital and was treated with a variety of antibiotics and cranberry capsules. After three weeks he still had the infection. There was some doubt if he would survive the infection. Finally it was decided to add DMSO to the treatment. He was given one teaspoonful of DMSO in cranberry juice three times a day along with the original antibiotic treatment. Improvement was rapid, and the patient returned home four days later with the infection completely under control.

When this patient returned home his care giver and the patient were advised that he should drink plenty of water along with cranberry capsules and DMSO. For his first week at home the patient was to take the DMSO twice a day. After the first week the DMSO was reduced to once a day. The infection did not return, and the patients' mobility and overall health became better than it was before he suffered from the infection.

Chapter 22

Inflammation

Inflammation is a complex reaction of the body to injury or destruction of tissue that has been damaged by disease or injury. In the acute form it is characterized by the classical signs of pain, swelling, heat, redness, and loss of function.

Certain conditions such as arthritis can lead to chronic inflammation which increases the pain from the original problem. Acute inflammation can be caused by injuries, burns, infections, or any of a wide variety of illnesses or other causes.

As mentioned in other chapters dealing with specific ailments, DMSO is a potent anti-inflammatory agent. It can minimize all the symptoms of inflammation. In the clinics we have observed swelling in patients go down, felt localized heat cool to normal, and the patients often mention immediate reduction in pain.

DMSO also increases the effectiveness of cortisol. Cortisol, which is produced in the adrenal glands, is the body's own natural anti-inflammatory hormone. In a laboratory study it was found that DMSO helped protect cells against a variety of agents even when cortisol concentrations were drastically reduced.

Cortisone, which is a steroid, is often used as a replacement for the natural cortisol which the body produces. Steroid drugs, including cortisone, can be beneficial when used for short periods of time and in small doses. When used properly, steroids can save the life of a patient suffering from acute asthma or allergy. However, when used for a longer period of time, steroids can provide life threatening side effects. These include gastrointestinal bleeding, retention of fluids, mental problems, broken blood vessels, weakness, free radical formation, and suppression of the immune system.

Sometimes the side effects from treatment are worse than the condition being treated.

Non steroidal anti-inflammatory drugs (NSAIDs) have many of the same side effects as the steroid drugs. These drugs can be especially toxic to the stomach and intestinal tract, causing severe bleeding, pain, and other problems. They are used by millions of patients for the relief of pain and inflammation.

One of the big problems of over the counter NSAIDs is that they are often taken by people without a good reason to take them. These patients have some pain and see advertisements, but may not even talk to a doctor before trying the drug. Often these patients have no idea that the drug they are trying can have very serious side effects.

DMSO has proven effective not only as an anti-inflammatory agent, but also as a treatment for some of the side effects of NSAIDs. Dr. Aws Salim, one of the world's top authorities on free radicals, conducted research on using free radical scavengers to treat side effects of NSAIDs.[1]

This study involved 180 arthritis patients with erosive gastritis that was caused by NSAID treatment. Fifty eight patients were given DMSO orally four times a day while 63 patients were given allopurinol orally four times a day. The other 59 patients served as controls.

Endoscopic examination 48 hours after admission to the hospital showed that gastric erosions were still present in significantly more untreated patients than those treated. The erosions remained in 50 percent of the untreated patients compared to seven percent in those treated with DMSO and nine percent for those treated with allopurinol. Since the only similarity between DMSO and allopurinol is that they are both free radical scavengers, the conclusion was that free radical scavengers reduce the NSAID induced gastritis and stimulate healing of the gastrointestinal tract.

An orthopedic medical clinic in Newport Beach, California has treated many arthritis patients who had previously been treated elsewhere. Most of these patients were previously treated with cortisone, NSAIDS, or both. This clinic very rarely used these drugs. DMSO along with diet and exercise was used to treat all patients with arthritis or injuries.

Many of the new patients suffered from severe digestive problems. The doctors at this clinic were not familiar with Dr. Salim's studies. However, they observed that when patients were treated for problems such as arthritis, chronic injuries, bone or joint problems, stomach and intestinal problems also showed rapid improvement. Long term bleeding often stopped in a few days, and patients reported that their long standing abdominal pains had completely stopped. In some cases these patients had previously been told that they would have to learn to live with the pain and bleeding.

DMSO should probably be used for all inflammation problems. It is not only a potent anti-inflammatory agent, it is also one of the most potent free radical scavengers and instead of harming the gastro intestinal tract, it actually helps make it more healthy.

---

1. Salim, A. S., A New Approach to the Treatment of Non Steroidal Anti-Inflammatory Induced Gastric Bleeding by Free Radical Scavengers, Surg Gynecol Obstet, May 1993; 176(5) 484-90.

Chapter 23

Interstitial Cystitis

DMSO was first approved by the FDA for the treatment of interstitial cystitis in 1978. Prior to this time there was no really effective treatment for interstitial cystitis. Interstitial cystitis is an inflammation of the inner lining of the bladder. The symptoms are similar to cystitis, a more common infection caused by bacteria which can be successfully treated with antibiotics. However interstitial cystitis is not caused by bacteria and does not respond to antibiotic treatment. DMSO is now the generally recognized and approved treatment for this condition.

Interstitial cystitis can cause severe symptoms in the bladder leading to scarring, bleeding, and a decreased bladder capacity. There can be intense pain, especially if the bladder is allowed to fill close to capacity. The pain is usually greatly reduced after the patient urinates. Some patients feel that they must urinate as often as 50 times a day. This urge usually continues both day and night. The condition is estimated to affect several hundred thousand people, most of them women.

When approval was first given for the use of DMSO in the treatment of interstitial cystitis, the treatment called for the use of a catheter to instill the DMSO directly into the patient's bladder. Treatments are usually once or twice a week. Some patients have so much pain that the instillation method cannot be used successfully. When this happens, the patient can take the DMSO orally in juice or water.

Many doctors contend that oral DMSO is the best way to treat interstitial cystitis because it is so much easier on the patient. In the oral treatment, the patient usually drinks one teaspoonful of DMSO in cranberry juice once or twice a day. Patients often report nearly immediate improvement, and it is not necessary for the patient to see her doctor every day.

Other doctors combine the two methods. They may give a bladder instillation to begin the treatment. Then they have the patient drink DMSO every day to keep the treatment going.

A 38 year old lady in Las Vegas, Nevada, reported to the clinic with severe abdominal pain and blood in her urine. She needed to urinate approximately every 30 minutes, and she told the doctor that she was sure that she would be dead in a few months. She was sure that she had cancer. After a complete examination and tests this lady was informed that she did not have cancer. The problem was interstitial cystitis. She was treated with a bladder instillation of DMSO and told to drink one teaspoonful of DMSO twice a day in cranberry juice. This lady felt better almost immediately. Two months later her symptoms had completely disappeared. She had also complained about depression and aches and pains in various parts of her body. These were also gone, and she said she felt like a new woman.

A 54 year old Los Angeles man with prostate cancer was treated with radiation. He went to see another doctor with a problem of severe pain and a large amount of blood in his urine. An examination revealed that this man had radiation cystitis. The decision was made to treat him with DMSO as it was known that DMSO helps protect against radiation damage, and DMSO had already been approved for interstitial cystitis. He was told to drink DMSO in cranberry juice twice a day. A reduction in pain and bleeding was noted practically immediately. Some bleeding continued for a number of months, but one year later he had completely recovered from the radiation cystitis.

Both radiation cystitis and interstitial cystitis can be very serious problems for the patient. The evidence shows that DMSO should normally be the treatment of choice for both of these ailments. Since DMSO is not toxic, no harm is done if the patient has an entirely different problem. This is often the case. Interstitial cystitis is difficult to diagnose, and it is estimated that thousands of cases are misdiagnosed every year. When DMSO is used the patient can normally benefit even if the problem has no relation to the diagnosis.

Chapter 24

Legality of DMSO

Many doctors seem to be unaware that once a drug has been approved for one condition, it can also be used to treat other conditions. The approval does not just apply to the condition for which approval was requested and granted. Once DMSO was approved for interstitial cystitis it could be used for other ailments.

This legality was clearly established in a court case involving H. Ray Evers, M.D. The Food and Drug Administration alleged that Dr. Evers was illegally administering EDTA in the treatment of arteriosclerosis while the approved use of EDTA was only for the treatment of heavy metal poisoning. This case, which was entitled The United States of America vs H. Ray Evers. M.D., Civil Action No. 78-93-N dated June 27, 1978 in the Federal District Court for the Middle District of Alabama, Dr. Evers won a major victory not only for his freedom to use EDTA but for medical freedom in general in the United States.

The FDA attempted to obtain an injunction to completely prevent Dr. Evers from using EDTA or any other chelating agent to treat any of his patients. The FDA even wanted the right to have regular inspections of Dr. Evers' clinic to make sure that he was obeying all orders.

The court first decided that the legal issue was whether a licensed medical doctor could be prevented from prescribing or using a drug on his patients which has not been specifically indicated for the patient's condition.

Even though many doctors were of the opinion that chelation had not been proven clinically to help arteriosclerosis, the evidence submitted to the court indicated that there was benefit. The court ruled that the risks to the patient were minimal and the probable benefits exceeded the probable risks in the treatment.

The court ruled that the laws did not intend for the Food and Drug Administration to interfere with the medical practice between the doctor and the patient. The court further ruled that the FDA had no right to interfere with private medical practice by limiting the doctor from treating according to his best judgment. In summary the Federal Court decision in the Ray Evers case is that it is the right of the doctor to determine the medical use of any drug once that drug has been approved for any condition.

This writer knew Dr. Evers and considered him to be a real pioneer in certain phases of medicine. He always seemed to be most interested in what was best for his patient, and he was willing to try something new if he thought it would be of benefit. In many ways he was similar to Dr. Stanley Jacob, the father of DSMO.

Chapter 25

Lupus

DMSO has proven to be the most important, or one of the most important, products for the treatment of lupus. It does not actually cure the lupus but it greatly reduces the symptoms so the patient can live with the disease. It does seem to be more effective than cortisone, and DMSO does not have the side effects of cortisone.

Lupus is an inflammatory disease with a wide variety of symptoms that can vary from patient to patient. It can cause fever, skin rash, fatigue, and joint pain that is often similar to arthritis. It can also severely damage internal organs, especially the kidneys. Lupus can cause severe pain and lack of mobility for a period of time and then suddenly improve. This improvement is usually only temporary, and then the disease can come back even more strongly.

One Los Angeles area woman who has had lupus for over 10 years has been avoiding the severe and painful episodes with the frequent use of DMSO. She usually receives an injection every week of DMSO and vitamins and applies a lotion containing DMSO to painful joints. She had originally used other medications that did not control the pain and also had many harmful side effects.

When she changed doctors, the original doctor, who was considered to be a specialist in auto-immune diseases, warned her about changing doctors. He told her that the treatment she was trying was not proven and that he knew much more about lupus than the new doctor.

The original doctor also told her that she would suffer much more without the methotrexate that he was using on her. He was very surprised when she later told him that she would never again use methotrexate for lupus or any other problem.

Methotrexate is a chemotherapeutic drug that is used for cancer. While it may reduce some of the symptoms of lupus, the long term side effects can be devastating and actually increase disability. This lady is now working at a full time job. She has some mild symptoms of lupus, but no extreme pain. Her internal organs are all functioning normally and are not expected to fail. Her only side effect with the DMSO is the garlic like breath odor. She says she now feels the best she has felt in over 10 years and plans to live a long healthy life.

Chapter 26

Mental Illness

DMSO has been used to treat patients with severe psychiatric problems including schizophrenia, alcoholic psychoses, obsessive-compulsive neurosis, severe anxiety, and other mental problems for over 40 years.

A major DMSO study involving 42 patients conducted in Peru was published in the Annals of the New York Academy of Sciences.[1] This study involved 25 schizophrenic patients, four manic depressive psychotics, four alcoholic psychotics, four compulsive-obsessive neurotics and five patients with severe anxiety states. A control group composed of 16 patients with similar problems was established. The patients in the control group received the normal psychiatric treatment for their conditions.

Before starting the DMSO treatment the patients were taken off all previous medications for at least one week. They were given DMSO in 5 ml intramuscular injections at either 50% or 80% concentrations. Most of the patients started with an 80% injection two or three times a day. In the most disturbed patients up to five injections a day were administered. Patients showing mild symptoms were started on one or two vials of 50% DMSO. As their symptoms improved, all patients were put on a 50% solution of DMSO.

The results of this study showed that DMSO is effective in treating mental illness. It also showed that acute patients responded much better than chronic patients.

Of the 25 schizophrenic patients, 14 were acute and 11 were considered chronic. There was rapid and dramatic improvement in the 14 acute cases. The most noticeable effect was the reduction of the agitation state. This improvement started with the first few doses and was particularly the situation with the six catatonic-paranoid patients who entered the hospital in a very agitated condition.

The 14 acute cases were all discharged from the hospital in 45 days or less. Three of these patients made a complete recovery 15 days after admission to the hospital. One of the patients said "I have been out of my mind. I don't know what happened to me. I wonder what my children are going to say."

The 11 chronic patients consisted of four patients who were under conventional treatment as outpatients, but were hospitalized when necessary. The other seven chronic patients were in a very bad mental state and had been in permanent hospitalization for over six years. These seven patients had all been unsuccessfully treated with electro shock, insulin, and phenothiazine drugs for more than four years.

The four long term schizophrenics who had been repeatedly hospitalized had complete remissions and were discharged from the hospital. Their response to DMSO treatment was faster than with conventional treatment, and their hospital time was shorter than it had been with previous hospitalizations of these patients or with similar chronic schizophrenics treated with conventional therapy. The remaining seven chronic schizophrenics showed improvement with the DMSO treatment, but were still unable to leave the hospital.

The four patients with manic depressive psychoses were in the manic phase when treatment was started. They were in a state of psychomotor agitation for an average of 15 days with megalomaniac ideas, verbosity, fighting, and other problems. These four patients all showed great improvement in their agitated condition. They became calmer and greatly reduced their verbosity and megalomaniac ideas. The manic phase was shorter and less intense than it had been in the previous episodes treated with conventional therapy.

Two of the patients suffering from alcoholic psychoses had alcoholic hallucinations, and the other two were in a delirium tremens condition. All four had been previously hospitalized for the same condition. They all showed improvement from the start of treatment. Restlessness decreased after the first few days even though hallucinations remained longer. Later these symptoms decreased in frequency and intensity until they stopped.

The patients with obsessive-compulsive neurosis and severe anxiety responded positively with the DMSO treatment. The patients were calmer, ideas did not upset them as before, they were able to act in a more spontaneous way, and they were able to overcome their obsessive compulsions.

This study showed complete and lasting remission of acute patients with a variety of mental problems and chronic schizophrenics with acute episodes. Improvements in the 7 chronic schizophrenics who had all been hospitalized for over six years lasted from 1 to 4 weeks after completion of treatment. When treatment with DMSO was again given to relapsed patients, they responded with the same favorable results as in the original study.

A more recent case in the United States involved Aaron Petras of Santa Rosa, California, a patient with a severe mental problem that was treated with DMSO. He had been diagnosed as a paranoid schizophrenic with severe delusions. His biggest problem was the idea that his foot was buzzing and that this noise disturbed other people and even dogs and cats in the neighborhood. He was an adult who was being cared for by his mother and was only hospitalized when he had severe episodes.

One time when I was visiting Mr. Petras in his home a dog across the street started barking. Mr. Petras immediately said "My foot is buzzing. That is why the dog is barking. I am disturbing him." I then had him remove his shoe and sock and checked the foot with a stethoscope. I could hear a loud heartbeat. Then I had him listen to his foot with the stethoscope and asked him if this is the noise that he hears from his foot. He said that was the noise and that it was upsetting the dog. I explained to him that the barking of the dog caused the loud beat and that there was no way that the dog or any person could hear his foot without a stethoscope.

It was decided to use a combination of DMSO, GH3, and vitamin B-12 injections on Mr. Petras. Before starting the injections, Mr. Petras' psychiatrist took him off all psychotropic drugs for two weeks. She said they were not really doing him much good anyway as his condition had declined over the previous 10 years.

Injections were given three times a week, and improvement was immediate. Mr. Petras became more calm and less fearful. He became more alert and clear in his thinking and better able to cope with reality. When treatment was discontinued his condition gradually reverted back to a more active chronic paranoid schizophrenic state. Later injections gave positive results similar to the original treatment.

There was one important lesson to be learned from this case. When Mr. Patras was first diagnosed, no one listened to his foot with a stethoscope so no noise was heard from his foot. Many times there is some basis in what a mental patient says. The doctor should always listen to what the patient says and try to determine the basis for the belief of the patient. Even though the patient is mentally ill, it can be beneficial to the recovery of the patient if he realizes that there is some basis to what he may feel or hear.

Recommendations for Future Studies

DMSO has been proven to safely reduce the symptoms of mental patients with a wide variety of problems. It is a product that should be used in all mental hospitals. Too many patients are admitted to mental hospitals with no hope of real improvement. Many of these patients could be helped to enjoy a productive life outside the mental institution with the proper use of DMSO.

There is no reason not to use DMSO in all state mental hospitals. Since there are no fatal or harmful side effects, there is no risk. Various dosages could be tried along with combinations with various drugs and vitamins to find out what works best. There is no reason for elaborate studies. The studies can be very simple with the methods and procedures as well as the results published so that others can take advantage of the research.

Many states and other government agencies are running low on money and face a major cash flow problem. Housing mental patients in institutions consumes much cash that could be used for other purposes or returned to the tax payers. The proper use of DMSO could undoubtedly reduce the population of the mental hospitals by over 50%, thereby reducing the cost. Even more important, many of those who are now confined to institutions could become happy, free, productive people.

[1.] Ramirez, Eduardo and Segisfredo Luza. "Dimethyl Sulfoxide in the Treatment of Mental Patients." Annals of the New York Academy of Sciences, Vol. 141, pgs. 655-667, 1967.

Chapter 27

Mental Retardation

DMSO has proven to be very effective in the treatment of mental retardation. In some cases DMSO is used by itself while in others it is combined with amino acids, vitamins, or other products. The DMSO has also been administered in various ways including oral where the patient drinks the DMSO in water, juice or milk, by intramuscular injection, or by topical application.

One major well documented study was conducted in Chile on 55 children with severe mental retardation caused by Down's syndrome[1]. Patients with Down's syndrome, which is also known as mongolism or trisomy of chromosome 21, are born with three chromosome 21's instead of the normal two. Those with the extra chromosome 21 are mentally retarded, and until DMSO little could be done to help them.

The patients in the Chile study were given DMSO and amino acids by intramuscular injection. The vials for injection consisted of 5ccs of 5% DMSO along with 5mg of gamma aminobutyric acid (GABA), 10mg of gamma amino beta hydroxybutyric acid (GABOB) and 10mg of acetyl glutamine.

The children were divided into two groups, those under 3 ½ years old and those over 3 ½ years old. Of those under 3 ½ years 15 children received the treatment, and 13 of the children served as controls. In those over 3 ½ years old with the oldest being 14, 16 children received the treatment while 11 children served as controls.

For the children under 3 ½ years old the dosage of the 5cc ampule containing the 5% DMSO combined with the amino acids was adjusted according to body weight. Those that weighed less than 8kg were administered .5cc, those between 8 and 11kg 1cc, and those that weighed more than 11kg received 2cc. All of the children over 3 ½ years old received the entire 5cc ampule in each injection.

With the children who were less than 3 ½ years old, the injections were given every other day for 90 days. There was then a one month break without the DMSO. All the children received a minimum of three cycles of injections. During the one month break the patients were given capsules that contained GABA, GABOB, acetyl glutamine and arginine, but no DMSO.

The children who were more than 3 ½ years old received injections ever day for 20 days alternating with 20 days off. During their 20 days break they were given the amino acid capsules that contained GABA, GABOB, acetyl glutamine, and arginine, but no DMSO. They all received five series of 20 injections each for a total of 100 injections.

Both groups of children showed large advances compared to the control groups. The psychometric testing of the children under 3 ½ years old was figured in accordance with Gesell's development quotient. Those treated with the DMSO improved in all areas with the results summarized below:

Motor area: In the control group there was very little change with an average of 56 before treatment and 58 after one year. In 10 patients out of 13 the motor index did not change while it dropped in one and rose in two. In the DMSO treated group the beginning average was also 56, but after one year it was 72.

Adaptive area: In the control group the beginning average was 52 and at the end of one year it had declined to 49. The DMSO treated group started with an average of 50 which increased to 60 after one year of treatment.

Language area: The control group had an average of 56 at the beginning and 54 after one year. The DMSO treated group had an average of 52 before treatment which increased to 58 after one year of treatment.

Children over 3 ½ years:

Motor area: In the control group the motor index average before treatment was 34 while after one year the average was 36. In the DMSO treated group the motor index average was 38 before treatment and 49 after one year of DMSO treatment.

Language area: Both the speaking and comprehension of the subjects was tested. In the control group the speaking average was 21 initially rising to 23 after one year while in comprehension the average was 25 in the beginning and 34 after one year. In the treated group the average score for speaking was 27 prior to treatment and 37 after one year while in comprehension the average was 42 prior to treatment and 52 after one year.

Intelligence Quotient: The children in the control group began the study with an average I.Q. of 34 and had an average I.Q. of 33 after one year. Those treated with DMSO had a beginning average I.Q. of 29 and had an average of 40 after one year of treatment.

The treating doctors agreed that the DMSO amino acid therapy is a big advance in treating children with severe mental retardation. They also recommended increasing the number of children treated and extending the length of treatment time. In the treatment of other children not related to this study they administered higher doses and obtained better results. Finally they stated that even though they have not arrived at an ideal treatment, the DMSO-amino acid therapy provides progress in treating a condition in which there has been no other progress in decades.

In another study presented at the New York Academy of Sciences conference on DMSO 26 non-mongoloid retarded children in Argentina were treated with the same DMSO amino acid therapy used in the Chile study.[2] Thirteen of the children received the DMSO treatment while the other 13 served as the control group. The group ranged in age from 5 to 20.

The DMSO treated children received a 5cc intramuscular injection three times a week in a series of 20 injections with a break of 15 days between each series over a total treatment time of 180 days.

The results of this study were similar to the previous study. There was very little change in the control group children while the DMSO children all showed some improvement.

Billy King of Portland, Oregon, is probably the best known patient in the United States to be treated with DMSO for Down's syndrome. He was a patient of Dr. Stan Jacob at the University of Oregon Medical School (now Oregon Health Sciences University) beginning in the early 1970s.

He was treated with DMSO every day. His mother told me back in the 1970's that he drank the DMSO in milk every morning. Of course this is something that every child could do. It is a simple and effective treatment that costs very little and can have a very big gain.

The picture on the next page shows how Billy looked in December 1971 before he was treated with DMSO and also how he looked after one year of treatment and after two years of treatment. When treatment first started he was 14 years old and had the mental capacity of a 10 month old. He could walk and feed himself. However, he could not speak or understand what other people said to him. At the time of the third picture after using DMSO for two years he had the mental abilities of a seven year old. He could speak and understand what was said to him. He could write his name and identify 269 Peabody flash cards. As shown by the pictures he had lost his Mongoloid looks. He could also swim across a swimming pool

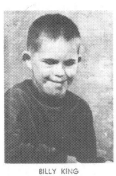

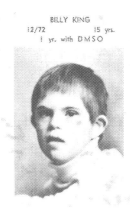

BILLY KING
12/72   15 yrs.
1 yr. with D M S O

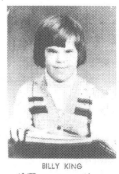

BILLY KING
12/71   14 yrs.
No D M S O

BILLY KING
12/73   16 yrs.
2 yrs. with D M S O

Billy King continued to improve over the years. As an adult he worked in a Portland book store. This is an example of someone whose life was completely changed with DMSO. He went from a person who had a very poor future, and who would have probably been dependent on others for support, to a productive adult who brought home a pay check every week.

What is the current status of the mentally retarded in the United States and other countries around the world? Many children who are like Billy King was before his DMSO treatment are in state institutions. Many, if not most of those who are severely retarded or who have suffered severe brain damage, could leave the hospital and lead normal lives. Your tax dollars are being thrown away in mental hospitals, and worse, patients who could be cured continue to be given tranquilizers to quiet them instead of DMSO treatment to cure them. It is time to start really treating these people and for those involved in the treatment to really believe that the severely retarded can be helped to become productive people.

---

1. Aspillaga, Manuel J,. Ghislaine Morizon, Isabel Avendano, Mila Sanchez, and Lucila Capdevile. "Dimethyl Sulfoxide Therapy in Severe Retardation in Mongoloid Children," Annals N.Y. Academy of Sciences 243: 421-431.

2. Giller, Ana and Maria E. M. de Bernadou, "Dimethyl Sulfoxide Therapy in Nonmongoloid Infintile Oligophrenia," Annals N.Y. Academy of Sciences 243: 432-448.

Chapter 28

Multiple Sclerosis

Multiple sclerosis is an inflammatory disease in which the myelin sheaths around the axons of the brain and spinal cord are damaged leading to demyelination and scarring. The disease reduces the ability of nerve cells to communicate with each other.

There are two general types of multiple sclerosis. One type is called the progressive form. This form generally disables and kills the patient more rapidly. The other type is called the remitting form. In this type there can be much recovery between attacks that damage the myelin sheath. Often patients with the remitting form live for many years. The recovery between attacks generally becomes less and less complete, and the attacks become more destructive until the patient dies.

Thirty four patients in Russia with multiple sclerosis were treated with DMSO as reported in a 1984 medical journal report.[1] The results were very positive in the patients who had the remitting type of multiple sclerosis. There was remyelination (growth of the myelin sheaths), a reduction in edema, and improved communication between the nerve cells. The improvement in the progressive type of the disease was not nearly as great as in the remitting type.

One patient in South Pasadena, California with the progressive form of multiple sclerosis was confined to a bed and a wheel chair. She was living in a convalescent hospital in a fetal position. Her knees were nearly up to her chest and it was not possible to move her legs. She was expected to be dead within a few months.

The family of this lady wanted her treated with DMSO, vitamins, and natural food. It was decided to give her intramuscular injections twice a week. She was given one teaspoonful of DMSO in water by mouth every day, and the nursing staff applied a lotion containing DMSO to her arms and legs every day.

Shortly after treatment started, this lady complained that the treatment was causing pain in her legs. Prior to treatment she had very little feeling in her legs so even this pain was considered to be positive. Slightly over a year after treatment was started, this lady was able to move her legs. She later was able to feed herself. Improvement continued until this lady was moved to another state to be closer to some members of her family who thought the same treatment would be available in her new location.

There was another interesting aspect to this case. The patient was on Medicare, and she needed physical therapy in addition to DMSO and conventional medical treatment. At first she was turned down by Medicare for physical therapy. A representative from Medicare explained that she had contractures and would never make much improvement. The situation was explained to the Medicare representative. He was told that she had already improved, and he was invited to visit the patient, review her medical records, and ask any questions he may have. He then agreed to reevaluate the case. However, he emphasized that the odds were against approval for Medicare reimbursement. After careful evaluation of the progress the patient had already made, she was approved for Medicare reimbursement for physical therapy.

This is another example of how any medical professional can often get other help that the patient may need. If you think the patient needs any treatment where reimbursement may be needed, and it has been denied, the denial should not be considered final. Often all that is needed is proof or a good indication that the proposed treatment offers benefits that exceed the cost.

1. Zingerman L. I "Dimexide (Dimethyl Sulfoxide) in the Treatment of Multiple Sclerosis Zhurnal Neuropatologii I Psikhiatrii Imeni SS Korsakova, 84 (9); 1300-1333, 1984.

Chapter 29

Pain

One of the major benefits of DMSO is its ability to greatly reduce pain. Pain comes in many forms and some problems that can cause severe pain are covered in other chapters. This chapter deals with pain in instances where pain is the primary problem.

Pain is basically an electrochemical warning from your body telling you that there is a problem. It is a warning to the patient that his body faces a potential danger that can cause, or is causing, actual tissue damage. DMSO can usually greatly reduce any pain. However, it is always best to find out what is causing the pain.

DMSO is not intended to replace the physician. If a patient has a persistent pain, there is a problem even if the cause of the problem is unknown. If the patient has appendicitis, the use of DMSO is not the answer. Medical advice and treatment should be obtained immediately. Surgery may be needed on an emergency basis to save the life of the patient.

Once the cause of the pain is known, DMSO can be used to the best advantage. Many times the best medical advice, examination, and tests fail to discover the cause of the pain. Also two people can have the same condition that looks similar on an x-ray, and one patient may have severe pain while the other patient has minimal pain. This can especially be true in back pain.

A patient in Newport Beach, California had suffered a severe back injury 10 years before first being seen at the clinic of Elmer Thomassen, MD. The patient had been involved in a major automobile accident and despite surgery had suffered from nearly constant pain since the accident. An examination showed some damage to the spine, but nothing in the area of most severe pain.

It was decided to treat this patient with a topical lotion of 90 percent DMSO. He was advised to have the lotion applied lightly to his entire back two times a day. The patient received some temporary relief after the first treatment. There was slight reduction of pain and less stiffness in the back. Treatment continued, and there was further improvement. After one year of treatment, the pain was nearly gone, and the patient had freedom of movement that he described as equal to what he had prior to the accident.

The patient was then advised to continue to apply the DMSO daily and to see the doctor every six months for examination and evaluation. The patient continued to improve. Two years after the original appointment he was hiking in the mountains, often walking over 10 miles on a Saturday or Sunday afternoon. He considered his general health to be better than before the accident. He said he would use the DMSO for the rest of his life and that neither he nor his wife objected to the smell of DMSO.

A controlled study involving patients with open chest surgery at Pennsylvania Hospital in Philadelphia showed excellent results in the control of post-surgical pain. In this study DMSO was applied to the 12-15 inch incision every six hours. Those receiving DMSO required only one half the normal amount of pain killers. They also had fewer complications such as nausea, vomiting, and constipation. They also recovered more rapidly from their surgery.

One of the worst pains that a patient can experience is a pain that is called phantom pain. This is a pain in a part of the body that is no longer there. An arm or leg may have been lost in an accident or the limb may have been amputated. However, it may feel to the amputee as though the limb were still there.

This phantom pain can be a burning or tingling feeling, a dull ache or very severe pain in all, or just a small part, of the missing body part. Sometimes the arm or leg will feel like it is getting numb, but it definitely feels like it is still there. The pain arises from various types of nerve stimuli which are not completely understood. The pain is real, not imaginary, even though the location of the pain is no longer attached to the patient. This pain is often difficult to treat.

A good example of phantom pain was a motorcycle rider in Los Angeles who had his right arm crushed in an accident. The arm was later surgically removed at his shoulder. This patient suffered pain that was mainly in his right elbow. At times the pain was sharp and severe and at other times he said it felt like the arm, especially at the elbow, was not getting a sufficient amount of blood.

This patient was first treated with DMSO in 1998, long after the accident. He had used a variety of pain medication, both over the counter and prescription, without any real relief. He considered most of his pain pills to be counter-productive as he said they provided more side effects that he did not like than pain relief that he did desire.

A lotion containing DMSO, capsicum pepper, and aloe vera juice was applied to the patient's shoulder at the amputation site. He made the comment shortly before the treatment that he was probably crazy to go for a voodoo treatment like this. He said: "You are treating me for a pain that is out in the air. The pain is not attached to my body. Maybe the pain is just in my mind. Nothing else has worked. I know this will not work either, but I am willing to show you that it won't work."

Minutes after the application of the lotion the patient said his arm felt better. He said: "I don't believe it, but my elbow feels much better. This stuff really works."

This patient was then advised to use the lotion twice a day whether he had pain or not. Three months later this man no longer had any phantom pain, and he was told that he could discontinue the treatment. The phantom pain did not come back. The patient used the lotion for other minor problems such as muscle aches and pains and said he would never again be without the lotion or plain DMSO which he drank in cranberry juice.

Any doctor who treats patients with pains of unknown cause, and this includes just about every doctor, should have DMSO available and know how to use it. Most pain medications have some potentially harmful side effects. With DMSO we have an effective and safe pain killer.

Chapter 30

Protection from Radiation Damage

The radio protective properties of DMSO have been known for over 40 years, DMSO has been used to prevent radiation damage from x-ray treatment and also to protect from high atmospheric levels of radiation such as that caused by accidents at nuclear power plants.

There is direct and immediate noticeable damage such as radiation burns. Radiation also produces free radicals that damage cells throughout the whole body. These free radicals cause the cells to age more rapidly and also cause the cells to mutate causing cancers, birth defects, and other diseases. DMSO is the most potent free radical scavenger known. Even low concentrations of DMSO can greatly reduce the radiation and free radical damage.

A study involving cervical cancer patients in Russia who received radiation treatment was reported in the Russian radiological journal Meditsinskaia Radiological.[1] In this study DMSO was applied topically to 22 cervical cancer patients prior to radiation treatment. The control group consisted of 59 patients who received radiation therapy without DMSO. The DMSO protected patients did not get radiation burns and other symptoms of radiation toxicity while the control group had the normally expected toxic reaction.

A study at Kyoto University in Japan involving the use of DMSO to protect DNA from radiation damage was reported in the Journal of Radiation Research in 2010.[2] In this study Chinese hamster ovary cells were exposed to radiation while being protected by a dilute solution (0.5%) of DMSO.

DNA is composed of two strands in the form of a double helix. It contains the genetic instructions used in the development and functioning of living organisms. The main role of DNA is the long term storage of information. DNA is often compared to a set of blueprints or plans since it contains the instructions needed to construct other components of cells. DNA can be from any organism such as a person, a dog, a cat, or a hamster. The DNA in hamster cells determines that the baby will be a hamster while the DNA in human cells determines that the baby will be a human. The DNA also influences the size, color, intelligence, etc. of the organism.

The DNA can be damaged in a variety of ways, one of which is exposure to radiation. Radiation can cause a break in some of the DNA strands. Previous studies by the Kyoto University researchers confirmed that a two hour treatment of irradiated cells with 10% DMSO could suppress deadly effects in the irradiated cells, but the concentration of DMSO was found to be toxic. The research showed that higher concentrations were effective in preventing double strand breaks. Generally the higher the concentration of DMSO, the fewer double strand breaks in the DNA, but since high concentrations proved toxic, the 0.5% DMSO was tried.

This study showed that 0.5% DMSO provided protection from radiation by helping repair double strand breaks rather than through indirect action of free radical suppression. Anyone who desires more detailed information on the Japanese study can access it on the internet. It is an excellent study even though it can be difficult to understand.

In their conclusion the authors of the study say that further studies are needed to truly understand the effects of DMSO in protecting the cells from radiation damage. Previously it was thought that the benefit was an indirect action caused by free radical suppression. However, as this study shows there is also direct action with the DMSO itself helping to repair the radiation damage to the DNA. There is still much to be learned about treating radiation damage.

How can the knowledge that we have now be used to help those who may have been exposed to an excessive amount of radiation, such as that from the damaged Fukushima Daiichi power plant? There were no previously written protocols for using DMSO in the treatment of radiation poisoning from damaged atomic power plants prior to 2011. The original protocols were written shortly after the Fukushima accident and should be considered subject to change as more information is obtained. However, it does provide a good basic starting point until more exact protocols are later designed. Also, the current treatment protocols can be varied to treat each individual case.

All of those exposed to excess radiation should be treated with DMSO immediately. The DMSO can be given by mouth, by injection, or by topical application to the skin. In some cases all three methods can be used. Those who have major exposure such as the workers at the power plant should be given heavy doses of DMSO. A maximum of 5 grams per kilogram of body weight on the first day is safe over a 24 hour period. However, this heavy dose is recommended only if the patient has received a massive dose of radiation that is considered to be immediately life threatening. Of course the patient should also be immediately removed from the source of the excess radiation. In the case of a nuclear power plant accident, this might mean that the patient should be moved 100 miles or more away from the accident site.

After the first day the dosage is greatly reduced. A permanent dose of up to one gram per kilogram of body weight can be taken by a person who is receiving a regular dose of excess radiation such as from a nuclear power plant accident or nuclear bomb. Protection from radiation is especially important for pregnant women. The DNA of the developing fetus is especially vulnerable to radiation damage. The result of radiation poisoning can be a deformed child, leukemia, or some other health problem.

Topical DMSO can be at a concentration of 90% for much of the body. Generally for the face the concentration should be 70% or less. It should be applied lightly at first to see how the patient responds. If the patient has radiation burns Scott Supreme Skin Lotion which contains 50% DMSO and also aloe vera has proven effective. Those that continue to receive radiation can apply DMSO or Scott Supreme Skin Lotion lightly on the whole body two or three times a day. The skin should be clean with no rubbing alcohol on the area where DMSO is applied as the DSMO can take other products with it through the skin.

When DMSO is taken by mouth, the concentration should be kept to 20% or less DMSO. The patient should drink the solution slowly after eating. Usually it is best to put the DMSO in juice to cover up the taste. However, it can also be diluted with water.

Other treatments can also be given along with the DMSO. These will not be covered in this book, but they include potassium iodide to help protect the thyroid if radioactive iodine is one of the contaminating agents. Epsom salt baths are also used along with other toxin reducing agents. Excess radiation can be obtained from many other sources that are not life threatening at the time, but can build up during the life of the patient. When the patient receives a diagnostic x-ray, the rest of the body is normally protected by a lead shield. If DMSO is applied topically to the area to be x-rayed, this will further reduce damage without harming the effectiveness of the x-ray.

DMSO has been used to successfully treat a wide variety of problems for over 50 years. It is considered to be one of the safest medicines ever used, and even though it has been used by millions of people there have been no documented cases of anyone ever having a fatal reaction to DMSO. The only side effect usually is garlic like breath. With topical use there may be some minor skin irritation which usually only lasts a few minutes. Anyone who receives a heavy dose of radiation from any nuclear power plant accident or other source should receive long term DMSO treatment to reduce the long term radiation damage.

1. G. M. Zharinov, S.F. Vershinina, and O.I. Drankova "Prevention of Radiation Damage to the Bladder and Rectum Using Local Application of Dimethyl Sulfoxide" Meditsinkskaia Radiologiia 20 : 16-18 March 1985

2. Genro Kashino, Youn Liu, Minor Suzuki, Shin-ichiro Masunaga, Yuki Kinashi, Koja Ono, Keiz Tano, and Masami Watanabe "An Alternative Mechanism for Radioprotection by Dimethyl Sulfoxide, Possible Facilitation of DNA Double Strand Break Repair" Journal of Radiation Research. Vol. 51, 733-740 2010

Chapter 31

Respiratory Problems

Respiratory problems severely affect the lives of many people both in the United States and in other countries around the world. These ailments can be especially deadly in infants and the elderly. DMSO, usually combined with other products such as antibiotics and anti-inflammatory drugs, has been proven effective in the treatment of most respiratory problems.

A study in Chile involving 60 babies with severe bronchiolitis shows the effectiveness of adding DMSO to the conventional treatment.[1] These babies were divided into two groups. Thirty of the babies were used as controls and were treated with antibiotics, oxygen and the steam tent. The DMSO group received the same treatment, but also an aerosol spray containing DMSO, an antibiotic and an anti-inflammatory drug. Those treated with DMSO had an immediate recovery. Thirty minutes after the DMSO treatment, 80 percent of the babies had sensorial and coughing improvement and 75 percent had decreased respiratory rate and improved breathing ability.

There was also a deferred benefit as the DMSO group did not require the use of the steam tent. The DMSO spray decreased the inflammatory process and the viscosity of the respiratory secretions so they could more easily be coughed up. The final conclusion of those conducting this study in their own words was "Since the application is easy, there are no toxic side effects and in view of the favorable results in the clinical evolution of the acute respiratory obstructive processes, we consider the use of this therapeutic spray very useful and beneficial in bronchiolitis.

One example of the children who were treated at this hospital was a three year old child who was very ill with a high fever, cough, and dyspnea. His condition continued to deteriorate, and he was given a tracheotomy 12 hours after his admittance to the hospital. Two days later he was transferred to the bronchopulmonary service where his general condition was considered deficient.

It was decided to give this patient one ml of DMSO spray by use of a tracheal cannula. He reacted by severe coughing and temporary suffocation, followed by the expulsion of a large amount of secretion. His breathing immediately improved, and he became calmer. He was discharged from the hospital nine days after he entered and was considered cured.

Asthma is considered to be the most common chronic illness of children. It is an inflammatory condition of the bronchial tubes. Excessive amounts of mucus develop. An acute asthmatic attack can make breathing so difficult that the patient can die from lack of oxygen. Asthma can affect people of all ages, not just children, and the condition can actually be more serious in the elderly.

The normal medical treatment for asthma has mainly centered on symptom reducing drugs. Inhalers are used to expand the air passages. Anti-inflammatory drugs are used to prevent the formation of mucus which can in extreme cases completely block breathing. Cortisone is often also used. While these treatments can be lifesaving in an emergency, they can have bad side effects, especially when used frequently and for long periods of time.

DMSO has been proven effective in treating asthma without the side effects of cortisone and bronchodilators. This is often done in a very simple manner such as topical application of DMSO either by itself or in combination with various medicines and herbs.

This writer has a great grandson that was a rather severe asthmatic as a baby. His mother took him to a doctor who prescribed the standard medical treatment at that time. This provided some relief as he was able to breathe a little better although not as well as desired. His mother was also concerned about toxic side effects of the medication.

Complete relief from his asthma was finally obtained by the use of a DMSO lotion. This lotion contained aloe vera juice and eucalyptus oil along with the DMSO. The lotion was applied on his chest, around his nose, and on his forehead at night just before he went to bed. He had immediate relief. He could breathe without difficulty. For a number of years after this he would not go to bed without his lotion. He has since quit using the lotion every night as he no longer has the asthma. Some children grow out of their asthma as they get older. However, it is possible in this case that once the cycle of the asthma was completely stopped by the lotion for a period of time, the asthma did not come back.

This example is just one of many that show that DMSO should probably be tried in the treatment of most respiratory problems. This does not mean that a person with asthma who is on other medications such as cortisone should stop that medicine suddenly after taking it for years. This can result in severe problems, even death. Some medications must be stopped slowly. This should be done only under the supervision of a doctor. When you take cortisone for a long period of time your adrenal glands stop producing cortisol, the natural cortisone hormone. You cannot stop cortisone suddenly. There are tests that can be given by the doctor to help determine how cortisone and other medications can be reduced and eliminated.

There are other natural things that can be done to help all respiratory problems. One of the most important is to keep the body hydrated. Water is the preferred drink. Coffee and alcoholic drinks do not count as liquids as they tend to dehydrate the body.

Allergies are often a prime or contributing factor in asthma and other respiratory problems. DMSO can help these allergies.

In fact some people who started taking DMSO for arthritis found that their coughing, sneezing and other allergic symptoms to pollen were stopped. Still the patient should also try to stay away as much as possible from any irritant. This includes food allergies, any pollen that may cause an allergic reaction, and tobacco smoke.

[1.] Zuniga, Aristides, Radolfo Burdach, and Santiago Rubio," Dimethyl Sulfoxide in Bronchiolitis," Annals of the New York Academy of Sciences, 243: 460-467

Chapter 32

Scleroderma

Scleroderma, an ailment of unknown cause which calcifies body tissue and can attack various internal organs, is a disease where DMSO is the only effective treatment. This condition affects over twice as many women as men and most often attacks those between 25 and 45 years of age.

The progress of this disease varies greatly from person to person. In some patients only the fingers may be affected for several years. Some patients suffer from scleroderma for over 25 years. Others die within a few years of diagnosis due primarily to organ failure caused by the disease. Seventy percent of the patients with systemic scleroderma die within seven years of diagnosis.

One of the largest scleroderma studies using DMSO was carried out at the Cleveland Clinic in Ohio where 43 patients were treated starting in 1965. These patients had been diagnosed as mild, moderate, or severe, and had suffered from scleroderma for from 1 to 25 years. They were treated with DMSO concentrations of 30 to 100 percent applied to various areas of the skin or even over the entire body.

Dr. Arthur L. Scherbel, who led the study, reported that this research provided the first time they had observed any positive changes in this ailment. After the patients had been treated for from 3 to 23 months, Dr. Sherbel and his group rated the progress made by each of the patients. Twenty six of the 43 had made good to excellent progress. Generally those showing the least symptoms showed the greatest improvement.

Only two patients whose scleroderma was far advanced scored good to excellent. Six patients with severe advanced scleroderma died during treatment or within three months of completing treatment. Neither those that died during treatment nor any of the other patients showed any harmful effects due to the treatment. Three patients stopped treatment after one year because all symptoms had disappeared, and they remained symptom free for at least six months of observation. Nine other patients discontinued treatment when their symptoms left, but pain and other symptoms recurred so they resumed treatment.

Other studies have provided similar results. Every study involving the treatment of scleroderma with DMSO with which this writer has knowledge has produced very positive results.

A more recent case involved a Santa Barbara, California woman who had suffered from scleroderma for many years. When she first started DMSO treatment, she weighed 79 pounds, bled from her kidneys, and frequently passed out. The prognosis was that the fainting spells would increase and eventually she would not wake up, unless she died of kidney failure first. She was in constant pain despite pain medication and was unable to work.

DMSO was applied on the arms, hands, feet and legs of this woman twice a day. She also drank a teaspoonful of DMSO in juice twice a day. She was also placed on an exercise program where she gradually increased her walking distance. She was given a diet that emphasized raw fruits and vegetables and no refined sugar.

Positive results were noted almost immediately. The pain was greatly reduced and she had more energy. Seven years later she no longer passed out or bled from her kidneys, and her weight had increased to 107 pounds. She had no scleroderma pain, was physically active, and seemed to be heading for complete recovery.

There has been no contact with this woman for a number of years. We assume and hope that her scleroderma stayed in remission. If the disease had come back there would most like have been contact in later years.

Chapter 33

Shingles & Herpes

DMSO has been proven effective in the treatment of viral infections, including the herpes virus. Results have been obtained with a combination of DMSO and various anti-inflammatory and antiviral medicines as well as with DMSO by itself.

Herpes zoster, more commonly known as shingles, can be especially serious. This disease comes from the same virus that causes chicken pox. The current theory is that the patient had chicken pox as a child and later in life, usually as a senior citizen, the virus is activated and there is an attack of shingles. Usually shingles will last up to a few weeks, and the patient then makes a full recovery. However, if the disease attacks the face, the shingles can get into the eyes of the patient sometimes causing permanent blindness.

When the sores of shingles disappear there can be a condition called postherpetic neuralgia. This can be extremely painful, and the pain can last for years. DMSO and other medications can reduce the pain of postherpetic neuralgia, but not eliminate it. One of the most important things in treating a patient with shingles is to prevent postherpetic neuralgia. It is much easier to prevent than to treat. The best way to prevent the neuralgia is to treat the shingles in its earliest stage.

A DMSO spray which also contained other antiviral and anti-inflammatory medicines was used by Lazano Sehtman, a dermatologist at Alrear Hospital in Buenos Aires Argentina, to treat patients with both herpes zoster and herpes simplex. Results were dramatic, all 17 cases of herpes (10 herpes simplex and seven herpes zoster) showed results within 48 hours with two applications of the spray per day.

Dr. William Campbell Douglas, an American doctor, had a clinical study of DMSO involving 46 patients with shingles in 1971. In this study he applied DMSO at strengths ranging from 50 percent to 90 percent on the skin lesions. Some of the patients received only DMSO while others had DMSO combined with dexamethasone. There seemed to be no difference in the results whether DMSO was used by itself or combined with the other drug. The best results were usually obtained on patients that were treated early in the disease process.

Some doctors, especially those that specialize in natural treatments, have used DMSO and lysine to treat both herpes zoster and herpes simplex. Lysine has been scientifically proven to retard the growth of the herpes virus and to inhibit viral replication. Usually up to 3000 mg of lysine is taken orally along with oral and topical DMSO.

It is usually more effective to both apply DMSO to the affected area and to give the DMSO by mouth or injection. Often the patient can be advised to take a teaspoonful of DMSO in water or juice three times a day. Topical DMSO can also be applied at strengths of 50 to 90 percent. The highest concentration possible that does not give the patient excessive pain is usually used. The topical applications can also be diluted with aloe vera juice instead of water. This can make the DMSO lotion even less painful.

All the studies and clinical results seem to indicate that early treatment is important to get the best results. The sores heal faster with DMSO when they have been present for a shorter time. Also postherpetic neuralgia can probably be completely prevented if DMSO treatment is started in the first few days of the disease.

Chapter 34

Spinal Cord Injuries

Severe back injuries, especially those involving the spinal cord, are often very difficult to treat by conventional methods. It is often impossible to know until later how much damage if any was done to the spinal cord by automobile accidents, industrial accidents, diving accidents, sports injuries, or other trauma.

Back and neck injuries present complex medical problems that often involve much more than the possible immediate damage to the spinal cord. These injuries also cause free radical formation, edema, decreased blood flow, and a lack of oxygen. One of the first things that happens after spinal cord injury is a reduction of oxygen and blood flow as the blood vessels constrict. Without proper treatment the tissue can then swell. This can lead to paralysis, either temporary or permanent, even if the spinal cord was not severely damaged by the original injury.

The unique properties of DMSO make it the most useful agent currently known to treat these problems. DMSO is the most powerful free radical scavenger known. It reduces edema, and it helps increase blood flow to the damaged area. The increased blood flow also increases the amount of oxygen and other essential products going through the injury site. Of course if the spinal cord is completely severed, there is currently no treatment that can relieve the damage. No surgery, DMSO, or other treatment can at the present time repair a severed spinal cord, and the patient will remain paralyzed from the point of severance down.

Usually the most effective DMSO treatment for spinal cord injury is by the intravenous slow drip method. Immediately after the intravenous injection of DMSO, there is an increase in the amount of blood flow in the area of the spinal cord injury.

The DMSO can also be given by mouth in juice or water, or it can be applied topically to the spinal area. DMSO treatment should be started as soon as possible after the injury. The longer the delay in treatment, the more likely there will be permanent damage. However, DMSO treatment, even years after the injury, can be better than no DMSO treatment.

An Orange County, California, engineer suffered a severe back injury in an automobile accident. He was paralyzed below the point of injury and was confined to a wheelchair. However, his spinal cord was not severed. It did suffer damage, but there was no break. DMSO treatment was offered, but this man refused the treatment. He was convinced that it would not work, and he would never walk because a few months after the accident he still had no feeling in his legs.

Twelve years after the accident this man changed his mind and decided to try topical treatment with a DMSO lotion. The lotion was applied twice a day to the entire back of this patient. After three months this man was able to move the toes on his right foot. He never regained the ability to walk, but the treatment restored some feeling and the ability to move a part of his body below the injury site.

Would this patient be able to walk if he had received DMSO in a timely manner shortly after the accident? No one can say for sure. However, this man now believes that if he had received proper DMSO treatment immediately following the accident, he would now be walking.

Any doctor in private practice can treat any patient with DMSO. It is often impossible to know at first the exact extent of an injury to the spinal area. There is never any danger in using DMSO even if the spinal cord is severed, and the patient is permanently paralyzed. If the patient has what appears to be a major injury, but the spinal cord is not severed, treatment with DMSO can sometimes lead to complete recovery by the patient.

Chapter 35

Skin Problems

A large study of 1371 patients in Chile with chronic skin ulcers was presented in the 1975 Annals of the New York Academy of Sciences.[1]

The skin ulcers were due to a wide variety of causes such as diabetic sores, infected wounds, and burns. The majority of the burns were infected. Many of the sores had been present for years and had been treated unsuccessfully with other medications.

This treatment consisted of DMSO mixed with antibiotic and anti-inflammatory agents. The mixture was sprayed directly on the wounds. In the majority of the cases, the treatment was given three times a week. In some cases of deep wounds, there was some pain at the time of application. However, this pain only lasted a short time and did not prevent treatment. Most patients received immediate relief and in some cases the pain completely stopped after the first treatment.

Dr. Mirando-Tirado said they were surprised by the rapid healing which occurred after only three treatments in some superficial infected wounds. Of the total number of patients 1313 (95.04%) were considered to be completely cured and able to resume their normal activities.

Several individual examples were given. One involved a 60 year old man who had been suffering from an ulcer of the right leg for 15 years. This ulcer which was two inches in diameter was caused by the rupture of a varicose vein. Various types of treatment had been tried over the 15 years that he suffered from the problem. However, nothing really worked. After 20 treatments with the DMSO spray, the ulcer healed completely and the sore did not return.

Another example given was a 55 year old man who had postphlebitic and hypostatic syndrome of the right leg with ulcerations and dermatitis following prolonged bed rest which was required as a result of an elevator accident. Because of the fractures the patient was in a plaster cast for 18 months and again for two months. During the following seven years he was treated by various dermatologists and was hospitalized several times at the University of Chile Clinical Hospital. Improvement was always temporary and the ulcers reappeared within a few days of discharge from the hospital. After only 10 treatments with the DMSO spray over a period of less than four weeks the ulcers healed completely and the patient was able to return to work and to walk without problems.

More recently a 90 year old lady in Los Angeles suffered from severe varicose ulcers in both legs. This lady, who was a retired school teacher, was afraid that she had cancer of both legs. It was explained to her that she had varicose veins. These later caused sores or ulcers to form. The dermatologist wanted to operate to remove the bad veins. This lady was treated with a skin lotion containing DMSO, aloe vera, and eucalyptus oil. The lotion was applied to both legs twice a day. There was immediate reduction of pain. One month later the sores were completely healed and have not returned.

How about skin problems of animals? A few years ago a cat in Los Angeles was having severe skin problems. The hair on a large part of her body was falling out. The skin was raw and bleeding. The owner of the cat took her to various veterinarians who tried a variety of tests and treatments. Nothing seemed to work, and it appeared the cat might be terminal. Finally a lotion containing DMSO was tried. Pain seemed to be reduced within a matter of minutes. The cat quit scratching herself. Her skin healed, and her hair grew back. Two months later she was a beautiful healthy cat. The treating doctor said he did not know what caused the skin problems, and he did not want to guess. However, he said that any future problems of that nature or any other skin problem of unknown cause suffered by another cat would first be treated with the DMSO lotion.

Skin grafts are sometimes needed following severe damage to the skin. They can be especially important when used in facial reconstruction. The biggest problem with these skin grafts is that survival of the grafts, except for the very smallest, is unpredictable.

A study was conducted by the Department of Otolaryngology-Head and Neck Surgery, University of Minnesota School of Medicine, Hennekin County Medical Center, Minneapolis, Minnesota on the effects of angiogenic growth factors and DMSO on composite grafts. In this study the angiogenic growth factors, basic fibroblast growth factor, and endothelial cell growth factor and DMSO were applied to grafts to determine their effects on vascularization and survival. This was administered either topically or by intradermal injection to 120 auricular grafts in New Zealand white rabbits.

Dermabrasion was performed in two groups in an attempt to increase transdermal delivery. The grafts were evaluated three weeks later and had a 40% increase in vascular ingrowth compared to the controls. An important discovery was that DMSO with dermabrasion increased graft survival even without an angiogenic agent.

DMSO can be the best friend of the dermatologist. Often a patient will come in with a skin problem of unknown cause. Sometimes extensive tests fail to reveal the cause. The patient can feel and see the problem. The doctor can see the problem and check for possible causes and not find the true problem. In these cases he can try DMSO by itself or with other products. Generally if the treatment does not provide relief, it will at least not harm the patients.

---

1. Miranda-Tirado, Rene "Dimethyl Sulfoxide Therapy in Chronic Skin Ulcers" Annals of the New York Academy of Sciences, Volume 243 pgs 408-411.

Chapter 36

Stroke

DMSO should probably be used in the treatment of all stroke patients. DMSO has a number of properties that make it valuable in treating any problem involving the brain.

One very important property of DMSO is the ability to cross the blood-brain barrier. It is one of the few products to cross this protective barrier. The blood-brain barrier serves as a protective mechanism that exists between circulating blood and the brain. It protects the brain from substances which are toxic to brain tissue.

There is normally an accumulation of water in the brain as a result of the stroke because the stroke damage breaks down some of the cells. The fluid buildup in the cranium compresses other brain cells resulting in the death of more cells. DMSO actually helps to remove the excess fluid from the brain resulting in lower pressure and less brain damage. There can also be an accumulation of blood that should be removed if it is providing pressure on brain cells. The best way to remove this blood is through the use of DMSO. The DMSO helps other blood vessels take over the work of the damaged blood vessels, thereby potentially saving the life of the stroke victim.

DMSO also protects nerve cells from any disruption following stroke injury. Other products have been used for this, but DMSO provides better protection than the other products. Another important consideration is the fact that there are no harmful side effects when using DMSO. The proper use of DMSO could save the lives of many stroke victims each year.

When the patient has a stroke DMSO treatment should start as soon as possible. Emergency personnel should all be trained in the use of DMSO. Ambulance crews should at least give DMSO treatment topically to all stroke patients when the patient is first picked up. When the patient arrives at the hospital he can have DMSO added to his intravenous infusion. Delay in starting treatment can result in permanent brain damage or death.

Immediate treatment is desirable even if the stroke is relatively minor. With a minor stroke immediate DMSO treatment will minimize the possibility of any permanent damage. If it is a major stroke immediate treatment with DMSO can often prevent major permanent disability or death. Brain tissue is very fragile and deteriorates rapidly if it is deprived of oxygen. When treatment is delayed certain brain functions can be destroyed permanently or the patient can die.

Even though early treatment is desirable good results have been obtained when treatment is started long after the stroke. A good example of a patient who was not treated immediately is a lady in Eugene, Oregon who did not receive DMSO treatment until three months after her stroke. This lady was in a coma in a convalescent hospital and had been in the coma since her stroke. She was given little chance of recovery and was expected to remain in a vegetative state until her death.

When I first observed this lady, there was no response to any type of stimulus. She was alive, but appeared lifeless. It was decided that her treatment should be topical DMSO applied to her head daily either by her husband or by one of the nurses at the facility.

One month after the start of treatment, there were positive signs in the lady. Her brain was starting to respond to the DMSO. The treatment continued, and four months after treatment started this lady was able to return to her home. After her return to her home, this patient started drinking one teaspoonful of DMSO in a small glass of water each day in addition to the daily topical treatment. This treatment continued for a period of years.

Three years after the start of DMSO treatment this writer returned to visit this patient. At this time the lady was living a normal life, not the life of a stroke victim. She was able to look after the house and walked normally. The only lingering effect of the stroke was a slight speech defect. At this time she said that her memory was better than that of her husband who had not had a stroke and who was considered to be completely normal.

A Los Angeles school teacher had a major stroke shortly after the start of the Christmas break. She was unconscious on her living room floor. DMSO treatment was started immediately after the stroke. The DMSO was first applied topically to her head within minutes of the stroke. Less than one hour after the stroke she was given DMSO by intramuscular injection. This patient was never taken to the hospital for this stroke. A prominent surgeon who was a family friend told the husband of this patient that it was important to keep her out of the hospital. The surgeon said that even though the treatment was completely legal, it would be difficult to get approval to give the DMSO especially by injection at his hospital.

This patient made a dramatic recovery. She regained consciousness later in the day in which she had her stroke. Treatment continued for the next week. Each day she received two topical applications of DMSO, one intramuscular injection of DMSO, and two doses of one teaspoonful of DMSO in juice. Her condition improved each day. When school resumed after the first of January, this teacher was back in the school teaching the students as if nothing had happened during the Christmas vacation. She never even mentioned it to the other people at the school. She continued teaching until she retired. She retired healthy with no disability.

DMSO has been known to be a superior treatment for strokes for many years. Some very well-known people have died needlessly of stroke. A good example was former president Richard Nixon who died four days after a major stroke. His final cause of death was listed as swelling of the brain. The swelling could have been prevented with the proper use of DMSO. Many years before Nixon's stroke, Dr. Stanley Jacob at Oregon Health Sciences University had been treating strokes with DMSO. The DMSO would have prevented the swelling. This writer remembers when it was announced that Mr. Nixon had swelling of the brain and had only a short time to live. At that time I said that his life could have definitely been saved if he had been treated immediately after the stroke. I also said that even though the swelling had started, there was still the possibility of reversing the condition with intravenous DMSO. Even topical application to the head might have been beneficial. However, DMSO was never used and a former president died without medical treatment that would have probably saved his life.

Chapter 37

Tooth & Gum Disease

Periodontal disease is the leading cause of tooth loss in middle aged and elderly people. It is a disease of the supporting structures of the teeth such as the gums, the periodontal membrane, and the bones supporting the teeth. It is generally caused by poor oral hygiene and a bad diet that often includes an excess of refined sugars. This encourages the growth of bacteria. Regular brushing with DMSO greatly reduces the bacteria growth.

Gum and supporting tissue disease goes through a process that in the earlier stages is called gingivitis. This is an inflammatory condition of the gums. Bacteria feed on food particles around the gums causing the formation of plaque which is composed of thousands of living bacteria. This forms in the gingival, the space between the tooth and the gum. The gums become swollen and bleed. If not properly treated, the plaque spreads to the underlying membrane and bone which can be severely damaged.

At this stage gingivitis becomes periodontitis. There is a progressive infection and more inflammation. The teeth become loosened and can fall out. If the process has not developed too far dentists can still save some loose teeth, especially if DMSO is used.

The bacteria have to eat to survive. They live on food particles left in the mouth after the patient eats. The bacteria also have to eliminate wastes, disposing of fecal matter on the teeth and gums. This is what causes the foul odor from the mouth of a person with gum disease.

The bacteria causing the plaque reproduce, and if left for a period of time die off. Dead plaque hardens and calcifies and is then called calculus or tarter. When the tarter builds up around the teeth, it causes the gums to pull away from the teeth. When this happens it creates a space allowing more food particles to accumulate causing even more bacteria. This also allows bacteria to enter the bloodstream. Studies have shown that heart disease is nearly twice as high in people with gum disease as it is for those with healthy gums.

DMSO has been used successfully in the treatment of tooth and gum problems since the 1960s. An official study in Poland involved 32 patients with periodontal disease.[1] These patients had inflammation and bleeding of the gums. In 13 of the patients the disease only involved bleeding and swollen gums. In the other 19 the infection extended deep into the gum, sometimes involving bone and loose teeth.

First the teeth were cleaned and as much bacteria as possible was removed. Then the patients were treated with compresses containing 30 percent DMSO for 10 minutes every other day for seven to ten treatments.

Great improvement was reported in all patients with superficial disease. Pain was eliminated, bleeding was greatly reduced and loose teeth became tighter in all patients. All patients with deep infections had less inflammation and less pain. Very loose teeth did not tighten up in any of the patients.

All periodontal disease should be treated by a dentist as soon as possible. Treatment is much easier in the earliest stages, and the results are much better. Loose teeth can tighten if they are not very loose. However, the use of DMSO has not, to this writer's knowledge, ever caused very loose teeth to tighten.

Many people use a 50 percent solution of DMSO as a mouth wash. Others brush their teeth with DMSO. This writer has brushed his teeth with DMSO for over 40 years with good results. His teeth and gums have caused much less problems since he started using the DMSO regularly. Other people apply DMSO when they have a tooth ache to relieve pain until the dentist is seen.

Some dentists regularly use DMSO in their dental practices to solve a number of pain, infection, and swelling problems. It is used both by itself and in combination with antibiotics and other medications. It is especially useful in treating the gum after extractions of teeth. The DMSO reduces swelling and pain and also reduces the risk of infection. Topical DMSO can also be applied to the external surface or the cheek or jaw next to the extraction site. One dentist in New York (Probably many more dentists also do this) uses DMSO to reduce radiation damage from dental x-rays. He applies DMSO topically to the area to be x-rayed shortly before the pictures are taken. Of course he also uses the normal lead protection normally used by all dentists.

The regular use of DMSO by the dentist and his patient can prevent many dental problems from developing. If a problem is present the DMSO can be used to reduce this problem. Teeth should last a life time. With the proper use of DMSO the patient is much more likely to live a long life with healthy teeth and gums.

---

1. Krzywicki, J. Czas Stomat, 1969, 1007-10.

Chapter 38

Toxicology of DMSO

DMSO has long been considered to be one of the safest products ever used in medicine. There have been no documented cases of death or serious injury from the use of DMSO even though millions of people have used it in the United States and in other countries around the world.

Despite the record of extreme safety clinical testing of DMSO was stopped in the United States on November 11, 1965 by the FDA. Dogs, rabbits, and pigs that were given massive doses of DMSO developed changes in the lens of their eyes. These changes were reversible and the lens became normal when treatment was stopped. It is noted that this problem did not occur in monkeys or more importantly in humans. However, at this time DMSO gained an underserved reputation of extreme toxicity. This continued until the Vacaville toxicology studies which proved the extreme safety of DMSO.

Two major studies on the toxicology of DMSO were conducted at the Vacaville, California State Prison Hospital in 1967 and 1968. These studies were divided into a short term study and a long term study. The short term study was conducted in October, 1967, and the long term study from November 21, 1967 to February 20, 1968.

These studies conducted using 80% DMSO topically applied to the skin at a rate of one gram per kilogram of body weight each day. This was from 3 to 30 times the estimated normal human treatment dose. Volunteers selected were healthy male inmates between the ages of 21 and 55. These men were all given a complete physical examination to make sure that they had no preexisting ophthalmologic, hematologic, pulmonary, renal, cardiac or hepatic ailments. Emotionally unstable inmates were not included in order to minimize distortion of any side effects.

The short term study was for 14 days. It consisted of 65 subjects who received DMSO and 33 subjects in a control group who received no DMSO. Blood and urine samples were taken from all subjects 7 and 14 days after the start of the treatment. At the end of the study all subjects also received a physical examination identical to the exam given prior to the treatment. The physical examination covered blood pressure, respiration, pulse, temperature, urinary and rectal systems, lungs, heart, eyes, ears, nose, throat, liver, kidney, spleen, skin, extremities, and neurology.

A complete ophthalmological exam was done at the end of the 14 day study and again two weeks after treatment and four weeks after the end of the treatment. The exam consisted of a complete testing of refraction and vision fields and an exam with the slit lamp and ophthalmoscope. The ophthalmological examination showed no significant negative changes such as those that had occurred in previous animal studies.

The physical examination did not indicate any problems. There was some skin drying and scaling, but all the skin returned to normal within three weeks of the end of treatment. The systolic blood pressure was slightly reduced in some of the patients, but this was not considered to be a problem. The final conclusion was that no serious side effects were observed in this study. Of course the garlic like odor of DMSO was observed in all patients.

The 90 day study was conducted in the same manner as the shorter study. Forty patients completed the 90 day study on DMSO and 16 patients served as controls. Tests and test results were similar in the two studies.

According to these studies where DMSO was given at 3 to 30 times the usual treatment dose for humans DMSO appears to be an extremely safe medication for human use. Most importantly, this study showed that the changes in the lens of the eye that occurred in certain animal species did not occur in man in this high dose, long lasting study.

What about the use of DMSO during pregnancy? There have been no official studies of which this writer has any knowledge. However, women have used DMSO while pregnant for the sole purpose of having a superior child. One of these was a nurse at Cedars Sinai Hospital in Los Angeles. Her child was much smarter than average. Another was a well-known author whose wife used DMSO every day while pregnant. Again the child was above average. While these two examples do not prove that the use of DMSO leads to smarter, healthier children, it definitely did not harm these children.

While I am not a doctor there are certain circumstances where I would advise my grandchildren to use DMSO during pregnancy. If my granddaughter were exposed to heavy radiation, such as from a nuclear power plant accident, I would definitely advise the daily use of DMSO throughout the pregnancy.

What are the long term risks of taking DMSO for a period of many years? No double blind studies of this use have been made. However, people have used DMSO for over 40 years with no observed side effects.

This writer first used DMSO in 1964 and has used it nearly every day for the last 49 years. During this time he has used it topically and taken it by mouth thousands of times. He now brushes his teeth daily with DMSO. He has also received hundreds of injection of DMSO. At 76 years old he has lived longer than the average age of both his parents and grandparents. He is the oldest of four children, three of whom are still living. He is the only one without any age related health problems. He also has a full head of hair which has retained its natural brown color. He is a top runner in his age group and uses a DMSO compound prior to any race.

Stan Jacob, MD, the father of the medical use of DMSO, is now near 90. He still works long hours doing medical research and writing. Most men his age who are still alive quit working many years before they reached 80. He is one of the few people in the world who has probably consumed more DMSO in his life than this writer. These examples show no long term toxicity in the use of DMSO.

Does long term use of DMSO increase human life expectancy? We do not know for sure, but the answer is probably it does. DMSO is a potent free radical scavenger, and free radicals contribute to the aging process so there is evidence that the regular use of DMSO can actually extend the life of the average person.

Chapter 39

Conclusion

DMSO has proven to be one of the most important products ever for the relief of human suffering. It is useful either by itself or in combination with other products in the treatment of nearly every ailment from which one may suffer. It has also been proven to be extremely safe. Despite the fact that DMSO has been used by millions of people, there have been no documented cases of death or extreme toxic reactions to DMSO.

Every doctor should become knowledgeable about DMSO. Its use can be incorporated into any type of medical practice. Often the doctor does not know what is wrong with a patient. Symptoms may be vague and tests inconclusive. However, it is known that something is definitely wrong. Under these circumstances, DMSO is often useful. It is very unlikely to do any harm.

Some medical authorities have pointed out that there is difficulty in performing double blind studies involving DMSO. The distinctive garlic like breath of those who use it often makes double blind studies impossible. There is an easy way around this problem. A group of patients can be compared with the results of untreated patients or those patients treated with the most commonly used treatments. If, for example, the normal treatment helps 50 per cent of the patients, but 80 per cent have undesirable side effects while the new treatment has the same effectiveness but no harmful side effects, the new treatment is definitely better. The placebo effect is often greatly exaggerated. Usually there is no reason for a patient or a doctor to automatically think one treatment is better than another unless it actually is better.

Since DMSO has so many medical uses, it does not fit into the idea that a medicine or treatment should just be for a specific ailment. Some doctors and regulators have a problem with a medication that helps a widely diverse range of problems.

Medical treatment is constantly changing. In the early years of the United States highly regarded doctors bled their patients with the idea of getting rid of bad blood. In many cases this bleeding led to death of the patient. Years ago sailors that used limes, lemons, and oranges to prevent scurvy were ridiculed by some members of the medical establishment. They thought it was crazy that vitamin C could prevent a serious disease like scurvy. They also pointed out that these sailors were not doctors, so they knew nothing about medicine.

DMSO is not the only treatment that has been mostly ignored in the United States. Homeopathic medicine is also now not generally accepted even though it has been proven to be safe and effective.

A number of years ago this writer read a book entitled Great Men of Medicine. This is a book that should be read by every medical student. The men and women mentioned in this book presented ideas, medicines, and treatments that were often ridiculed. The doctors were often persecuted because they had truths that conflicted with established errors and treatments. Often it was not until many years after their death that the contributions of these men and women were finally recognized.

Governments at all levels are in bad financial shape. In the United States Medicare payments could eventually bankrupt the country. State and county medical facilities spend too much money for too little results. If all these agencies properly utilized DMSO, results would be better and much tax money would be saved.

When DMSO is finally used as widely as it should, people throughout the world will be able to enjoy healthier, happier lives at a much lower cost for medical care.

About the Author

Archie Scott is a 1959 graduate of the School of Science at Oregon State University. Mr. Scott was first introduced to DMSO in 1964. He had suffered a major injury to his right knee in basketball in January, 1955, during his senior year of high school. Over eight years later in October, 1963, his left knee was injured in football. Despite surgery and other medical treatments both knees were taped during any athletic competition.

Starting in early 1964 DMSO was applied to both knees with good results. Pain was greatly reduced, and he was able to run much better.

He first met Dr. Stanley Jacob M.D., the father of DMSO, in 1966 and was placed on the mailing list of the University of Oregon Medical School (now Oregon Health Sciences University) from which he received information on DMSO and other medications for a number of years. This led to contacts with other doctors both in the United States and other countries. Even though he is not a doctor and has never claimed to be one, the knowledge he obtained led Mr. Scott to become a recognized authority on the medical use of DMSO.

Archie has served as a consultant to doctors and clinics in California, Oregon, Nevada, Florida, Minnesota, New York, and Mexico for over 40 years.